ANATOMY & PHYSIOLOGY SUPER REVIEW®

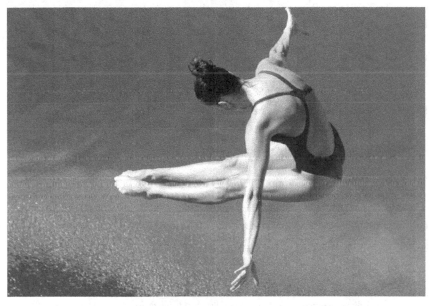

Jay M. Templin, Ed.D.
Professor of Biology
Former Science Coordinator
Montgomery County Community College
Pottstown, Pennsylvania

Research & Education Association
Visit our website at: www.rea.com

Research & Education Association
61 Ethel Road West
Piscataway, New Jersey 08854
E-mail: info@rea.com

ANATOMY & PHYSIOLOGY SUPER REVIEW®

Published 2016
Copyright © 2014 by Research & Education Association, Inc.
Prior edition copyright © 2000 by Research & Education
Association, Inc. All rights reserved. No part of this book
may be reproduced in any form without permission of the
publisher.

Printed in the United States of America

Library of Congress Control Number 2013932760

ISBN-13: 978-0-7386-1122-8
ISBN-10: 0-7386-1122-0

LIMIT OF LIABILITY/DISCLAIMER OF WARRANTY: Publication of this work is for the
purpose of test preparation and related use and subjects as set forth herein. While every effort has
been made to achieve a work of high quality, neither Research & Education Association, Inc.,
nor the authors and other contributors of this work guarantee the accuracy or completeness of
or assume any liability in connection with the information and opinions contained herein and
in REA's software and/or online materials. REA and the authors and other contributors shall in
no event be liable for any personal injury, property or other damages of any nature whatsoever,
whether special, indirect, consequential or compensatory, directly or indirectly resulting from
the publication, use or reliance upon this work.

All trademarks cited in this publication are the property of their respective owners.

Cover image: © iStockphoto/Thinkstock

SUPER REVIEW® and REA® are registered trademarks
of Research & Education Association, Inc.

H15

REA's *Anatomy & Physiology Super Review*®

Need help with Anatomy and Physiology? Want a quick review or refresher for class? This is the book for you!

REA's *Anatomy & Physiology Super Review*® gives you everything you need to know!

This *Super Review*® can be used as a supplement to your high school or college textbook, or as a handy guide for anyone who needs a fast review of the subject.

- **Comprehensive, yet concise coverage** – review covers the material that is typically taught in a beginning level anatomy and physiology course. Each topic is presented in a clear and easy-to-understand format that makes learning easier.

- **Questions and answers for each topic** – let you practice what you've learned and build your knowledge of the material.

- **End-of-chapter quizzes** – gauge your understanding of the important information you need to know, so you'll be ready for any anatomy and physiology question on your next quiz or test.

Whether you need a quick refresher on the subject, or are prepping for your next test, we think you'll agree that REA's *Super Review*® provides all you need to know!

Contents

About REA

Founded in 1959, Research & Education Association (REA) is dedicated to publishing the finest and most effective educational materials—including study guides and test preps—for students in middle school, high school, college, graduate school, and beyond.

Today, REA's wide-ranging catalog is a leading resource for students, teachers, and other professionals. Visit *www.rea.com* to see a complete listing of all our titles.

Acknowledgments

We would like to thank Pam Weston, Publisher, for setting the quality standards for production integrity and managing the publication to completion; Larry B. Kling, Vice President, Editorial, for supervision of revisions and overall direction; Kelli Wilkins, Copywriter, for coordinating development of this edition; PreMedia Global, for their editorial review and revisions; Ellen Gong for proofreading; and Christine Saul, Senior Graphic Designer, for typesetting this edition and designing our cover.

Available Super Review® Titles

ARTS/HUMANITIES
Basic Music
Classical Mythology
History of Architecture
History of Greek Art

BUSINESS
Accounting
Macroeconomics
Microeconomics

COMPUTER SCIENCE
C++
Java

HISTORY
Canadian History
European History
United States History

LANGUAGES
English
French
French Verbs
Italian
Japanese for Beginners
Japanese Verbs
Latin
Spanish

MATHEMATICS
Algebra & Trigonometry
Basic Math & Pre-Algebra
Calculus
Geometry
Linear Algebra
Pre-Calculus
Statistics

SCIENCES
Anatomy & Physiology
Biology
Chemistry
Entomology
Geology
Microbiology
Organic Chemistry I & II
Physics

SOCIAL SCIENCES
Psychology I & II
Sociology

WRITING
College & University Writing

CHAPTER 1

Introducing the
Human Body

1.1 Anatomy and Physiology

Anatomy - Anatomy is the study of the structure of body parts. It is also the study of the relationship among these parts. The heart, for example, consists of chambers, valves, and associated blood vessels.

Physiology - Physiology is the study of the function of body parts. The parts of the heart, for example, work together to pump the blood throughout the body.

There is a close association between anatomy and physiology. Structure complements function. The four chambers of the heart have muscular walls that contract to pump the blood. The makeup of the valves prevents the backflow of blood.

1.2 Levels of Organization

The anatomy of the human body is composed of different levels of organization. These levels represent a series of steps. Each level is a building step for the next level.

These levels are:

Atom - All matter consists of elements. These simple substances exist as discrete, submicroscopic particles called atoms. The four most common elements of the human body are carbon, hydrogen, oxygen, and nitrogen.

Molecule - Atoms bond into molecules. About 65 percent of human body weight consists of water molecules. Smaller molecules bond into larger molecules that have biological functions. Monosaccharides (e.g., glucose), for example, bond into polysaccharides (e.g., starch). These carbohydrates are an energy source.

Organelle - Molecules compose the parts of the cell called organelles. Each of these parts carries out a specific function. The ribosome, for example, is the site of protein synthesis.

Cell - The cell is the smallest unit displaying the properties of life. Cells tend to specialize. There are about 200 different kinds of specialized cells in the human body. Neurons (nerve cells) send signals. Leukocytes (white blood cells) fight infection.

Tissue - Similar cells function together in a tissue. Muscle cells work together in skeletal muscle tissue. These cells contract, producing body movement.

Organ - Two or more tissues work together in an organ. The heart is an organ that consists of several tissue types.

Organ Systems - Organs with related functions are part of the same organ system. The heart and blood vessels are organs of the circulatory system. They function to circulate the blood throughout the body.

Organism - All organ systems make up the organism. The organ systems of the human body include the nervous, circulatory, respiratory, and digestive systems.

1.3   Anatomical Terms

Anatomical terms are used to describe the makeup of the body accurately and concisely. All of these terms are used with reference to anatomical position. In this position the subject studied is facing forward and standing erect. The arms are hanging at the sides. The palms and toes are pointed forward.

1.3.1   Directional Terms

Directional terms compare the relative position of one body part to another body part. These terms occur in pairs. The members of each pair have opposite meanings.

Superior/Inferior - Superior means closer to the head. Inferior means closer to the feet. The neck is superior when compared to the chest, which is inferior. When compared to the abdomen, the chest is superior and the abdomen is inferior.

Anterior/Posterior - Anterior (ventral) refers to a part that is closer to the front of the body. Posterior (dorsal) refers to a part that is closer to the back. The heart is anterior when compared to the vertebral column, which is posterior. When compared to the sternum (breastbone), the heart is posterior and the sternum is anterior.

Medial/Lateral - Medial refers to a part that is closer to an imaginary midline passing vertically through the body. Lateral refers to a part that is farther from this midline. The nose is medial when compared to the eyes (lateral). When compared to the ears, the eyes are medial. The ears are lateral.

Proximal/Distal - Proximal refers to a part of a limb that is closer to the trunk (torso) of the body. Distal refers to a limb part that is farther from the trunk. The forearm is proximal when compared to the wrist (distal). The wrist is proximal when compared to the fingers (distal).

Other directional terms include:

Superficial - Closer to the surface of the body
Deep - Farther away from the surface of the body
Parietal - Referring to the wall of a body cavity
Visceral - Referring to an organ within the body cavity

1.3.2 Planes and Sections of the Body

Imaginary incisions can be made through the body to study the internal anatomy. These sections represent imaginary planes.

Sagittal Plane - A sagittal plane passes through the body longitudinally, dividing it into left and right regions. A midsagittal section passes through the midline of the body.

Coronal (Frontal) Plane - A coronal plane passes through the body longitudinally, dividing it into anterior and posterior regions.

Transverse Plane - A transverse plane passes through the body horizontally, dividing it into superior and inferior regions.

These sections can also pertain to organs of the body. Sagittal, coronal, and transverse planes all pass through the heart.

1.3.3 Body Cavities

There are two main cavities of the human body, the dorsal cavity and ventral cavity. Each cavity is divided into subcavities.

Dorsal Cavity - The dorsal cavity consists of the **cranial cavity** and **spinal cavity**. The cranial cavity is formed by the superior bones of the skull. It contains the brain. The spinal cavity is formed by a series of vertebrae. It contains the spinal cord.

Ventral Cavity - The ventral cavity consists of **thoracic** and **abdominopelvic subcavities**.

The thoracic cavity is superior to the diaphragm. It is subdivided into a left and right **pleural cavity**. The pleural cavities contain the lungs. The **mediastinum** is the space between the pleural cavities. It contains the trachea (windpipe), esophagus, thymus gland, and heart. The heart is contained within a separate cavity of the mediastinum, the **pericardial cavity**.

The abdominopelvic cavity is inferior to the diaphragm. The larger abdominal portion contains the liver, gallbladder, stomach, small intestine, and most of the large intestine. The smaller pelvic portion contains the rest of the large intestine, bladder, and reproductive organs.

1.4 Organ Systems

Organs with related functions are part of the same organ system. These systems are:

Integumentary System - The skin and accessory organs comprise the integumentary system. This system protects and regulates body temperature.

Skeletal System - The skeletal system consists of the bones and articulations (joints). This system provides protection and support. Skeletal muscles pull on bones to produce movements. The skeletal system also stores minerals and produces blood cells.

Muscular System - The skeletal muscles contract to produce body movements. The muscles also produce body heat.

Nervous System - The nervous system sends signals throughout the body. The central nervous system consists of the brain and spinal cord. The peripheral nervous system consists of the cranial and spinal nerves.

Endocrine System - The glands of the endocrine system secrete chemical messages called hormones. These messages regulate processes such as growth and mineral balance.

Circulatory System - The circulatory system transports substances to and from body cells. The lymphatic system is part of the circulatory system. One of its functions is to protect the body from disease.

Respiratory System - The respiratory system distributes and exchanges gases between the body and external environment.

Digestive System - The digestive system prepares food molecules for use by the cells of the body.

Urinary System - The urinary system controls the composition and volume of the blood. It eliminates wastes.

Reproductive System - The male reproductive system produces sex cells. It transfers these cells to the female reproductive system. The female reproductive system produces sex cells and receives the male sex cells. It also provides the internal environment for the development of the embryo and fetus.

1.5   Homeostasis

Homeostasis is the maintenance of relatively constant conditions of the internal environment of the body. The internal environment includes the interstitial (or tissue fluid), which bathes the cells. This tissue fluid is formed from the blood. Characteristics that are controlled include:

Temperature - an average temperature is 37° C
Blood Sugar - an average blood sugar level is 100 mg per
      100 ml of blood
pH of the Blood - the average is 7.4

These characteristics are controlled by **negative feedback**. Receptors sense changes in the internal environment. Through signals from the nervous and endocrine systems, responses reverse the trend of these changes. For example, if blood sugar increases, the pancreas secretes insulin. This hormone signals responses that decrease the level of glucose in the blood.

If body temperature decreases, responses increase body temperature. One response is the shivering of the skeletal muscles.

CHAPTER 2

Chemistry of Life

2.1   Elements and Atoms

Element - An element is a substance that cannot be broken down into simpler substances by normal chemical reactions. The four most common elements of the human body are carbon, hydrogen, oxygen, and nitrogen (see figure on the next page). Elements exist as discrete, submicroscopic particles called atoms.

Atom - Each element consists of one kind of atom. An atom is the smallest particle that displays the chemical properties of an element. The three main types of subatomic particles of an atom are the **proton**, **neutron**, and **electron**.

Atomic Weight - The atomic weight (mass) is the total number of protons and neutrons in the nucleus of an atom. For example, the atomic weight of carbon is usually 12; for oxygen it is usually 16.

Atomic Number - The atomic number is equal to the number of protons in the atom. For example, the atomic number of carbon is 6; for oxygen it is 8.

Isotope - Isotopes are atoms of the same element that have a different number of neutrons. Isotopes have different atomic weights. Oxygen is one atom having isotopes with the atomic weights of 16 (8 protons, 8 neutrons) and 18 (8 protons, 10 neutrons).

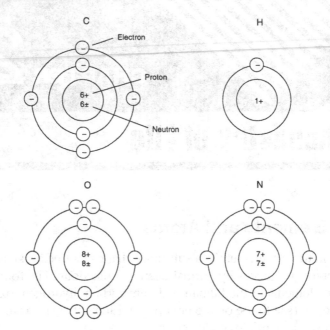

Planetary models of carbon, hydrogen, oxygen, and nitrogen

Ions - An ion is an atom that has lost or gained electrons. If the sodium atom loses its one outer shell electron, it becomes a positive ion (cation). If the chlorine atom gains one electron in its outer shell, it becomes negative (anion).

Problem Solving Example:

 Define the following terms: atom, isotope, ion. Could a single particle of matter be all three simultaneously?

Atom of helium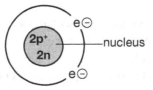

A An atom is the smallest particle of an element that can retain the chemical properties of that element. It is composed of a nucleus, which contains positively charged protons and neutral neutrons, around which negatively charged electrons revolve in orbits. For example, a helium atom contains two protons, two neutrons, and two electrons.

Isotopes are alternate forms of the same chemical element. A chemical element is defined in terms of its atomic number, which is the number of protons in its nucleus. Isotopes of an element have the same number of protons as that element, but a different number of neutrons. Because atomic mass is determined by the number of protons plus neutrons, isotopes of the same element have varying atomic masses. For example, deuterium (^2H) is an isotope of hydrogen and has one neutron and one proton in its nucleus. A hydrogen isotope has only a proton, and no neutrons, in its nucleus.

An ion is a positively or negatively charged atom or group of atoms. An ion that is negatively charged is called an anion, and a positively charged ion is called a cation.

A single particle can be an atom, an ion, and an isotope simultaneously. The simplest example is the hydrogen ion H^+. It is an atom that has lost one electron and thus developed a positive charge. Since it is charged, it is therefore an ion. Although they have different atomic masses, they must be isotopes of one another, because their atomic numbers are the same.

2.2 Water

About 65 percent of human body weight is water. A water molecule consists of two hydrogen atoms linked to one oxygen atom by polar covalent bonds (see figure on the next page). Its most important biological function is serving as a solvent for many kinds of solutes. A solution is a mixture of a solute and solvent.

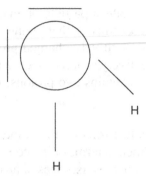

Structural formula of a water molecule

Acid - An acid is a compound that dissociates in water to yield hydrogen ions (H^+). An acid is a proton donor.

Base - A base is a compound that dissociates in water to yield hydroxyl ions (OH^-). A base is a proton acceptor.

pH - pH is a scale showing the degree of acidity or alkalinity of a solution. The scale has a range of 0 to 14. A pH of 7 is neutral. A pH of less than 7 is acidic. A pH of more than 7 is alkaline (basic). The skin, for example, has a pH of about 5. The pH of the blood is about 7.4.

Buffer - Buffers are compounds that stabilize the pH of a solution. They react to changes in pH if an acid or base is added to a solution.

Salt - A salt is a compound consisting of a cation other than hydrogen and an anion other than the hydroxide ion. One example of a salt is sodium chloride (NaCl). Salts dissociate into positive and negative ions (cations and anions) in water.

Problem Solving Examples:

 What properties of water make it an essential component of living matter?

A The chemistry of life on this planet is essentially the chemistry of water and carbon. Water is the most abundant molecule in the cell as well as on the earth. In fact, it makes up between 65 and 90 percent of the weight of most forms of life.

Life began in the sea, and the properties of water shape the chemistry of all living organisms. Life developed as a liquid-phase phenomenon because reactions in solution are much more rapid than reactions between solids, and complex and highly structural molecules can behave in solution in a way that they cannot behave in a gas. Water is an excellent solvent for living systems. It can stay in the liquid stage throughout a very wide range of temperature variation. Almost all chemicals present in living matter are soluble in it.

Water serves many functions in the human body. It dissolves waste products of metabolism and assists in their removal from the cell and the organism. Water functions in heat regulation almost as an insulator would. It has a high heat capacity or specific heat in that it has a great capacity for absorbing heat with only minimal changes in its own temperature because water molecules bond to one another by hydrogen bonds. Excess heat energy is dissipated by breaking these bonds, thus, the living material is protected against sudden thermal changes. In addition, the body uses water loss to cool itself. When water changes from a liquid to a gas, it absorbs a great deal of heat. This enables the body to dissipate excess heat by the evaporation of water. This process is known as sweating. Also, the good conductivity of water makes it possible for heat to be distributed evenly throughout the body tissues. Water serves as a lubricant and is present in body fluids wherever one organ rubs against another and in the joints where one bone meets another. Water serves in the transport of nutrients and other materials within the body.

Water is also very efficient in dissolving ionic salts and other polar compounds because of the polar physical properties of water molecules. The proper concentration of these salts is necessary for life processes, and it is important to keep them at extremely constant concentrations under normal conditions. These salts are important in maintaining osmotic relationships.

Differentiate between acids, bases, and salts. Give examples of each.

 There are essentially two widely used definitions of acids and bases: the Lowry-Brönsted definition and the Lewis definition. In the Lowry-Brönsted definition, an acid is a compound with the capacity to donate a proton, and a base is a compound with the capacity to accept a proton. In the Lewis definition, an acid has the ability to accept an electron pair and a base the ability to donate an electron pair.

Salts are a group of chemical substances that generally consist of positive and negative ions arranged to maximize attractive forces and minimize repulsive forces. Salts can be either inorganic or organic. For example, sodium chloride, NaCl, is an inorganic salt that is actually best represented with its charges Na^+Cl^-; sodium acetate, CH_3COONa or $CH_3COO^-Na^+$, is an organic salt.

Some common acids important to the biological system are acetic acid (CH_3COOH), carbonic acid (H_2CO_3), phosphoric acid (H_3PO_4), and water. Amino acids, the building blocks of protein, are compounds that contain an amine group ($-NH_2$) and an acidic group ($-COOH$). Some common bases are ammonia (NH_3), pyridine (C_5H_5N), purine , and water. The nitrogenous bases important in the structure of deoxyribonucleic acid (DNA) and ribonucleic acid (RNA) carry the purine or pyridine functional group. Water has the ability to act both as an acid ($H_2O \xrightarrow{-H^+} OH^-$) and as a base ($H_2O + H^+ \rightarrow H_3O^+$) depending on the conditions of the reaction, and is thus said to exhibit amphiprotic behavior.

 What does the "pH" of a solution mean? Why is a liquid with a pH of 5 ten times as acidic as a liquid with a pH of 6?

 The pH (an abbreviation for "potential of hydrogen") of a solution is a measure of the hydrogen ion (H^+) concentration. Specifically, pH is defined as the negative log of the hydrogen ion concentration. A pH scale is used to quantify the relative acid or base strength. It is based upon the dissociation reaction of water:

$H_2O \rightarrow H^+ + OH^-$. The dissociation constant (K) of this reaction is 1.0 $\times 10^{-14}$ and is defined as:

$$K = \frac{[H^+][OH^-]}{[H_2O]}$$

where $[H^+]$ and $[OH^-]$ are the concentrations of hydrogen and hydroxide ions, respectively, and $[H_2O]$ is the concentration of water (which is equal to one). The pH of water can be calculated from its dissociation constant K:

$$K = 1.0 \times 10^{-14} = \frac{[H^+][OH^-]}{[H_2O]} = [H^+][OH^-]$$

Since one H^+ and one OH^- are formed for every dissociated H_2O molecule, $[H^+] = [OH^-]$.

$$1.0 \times 10^{-14} = [H^+]^2 \ ; \ [H^+] = 1.0 \times 10^{-7}$$

$$pH = -\log[H^+] = -\log(1.0 \times 10^{-7}) = 7$$

A pH of 7 is considered to be neutral because there are equal concentrations of hydrogen and hydroxide ions. The pH scale ranges from 0 to 14. Acidic compounds have a range of 0 to 7, and basic compounds have a range of 7 to 14.

 What significance do buffers have in the living cell?

A buffering system is one that will prevent significant changes in pH upon addition of excess hydrogen or hydroxide ion to the body. Buffering systems are of great importance in the maintenance of the cell. For example, the enzymes within a cell have an optimal pH range, and outside this range, enzymatic activity will be sharply reduced. If the pH becomes too extreme, the enzymes and proteins within the cell may be denatured, which would cause cellular activity to drop to zero and the cell would die; therefore, a buffering system is essential to the existence of the cell. The average pH of a cell is 7.2, which is slightly on the basic side.

A buffer will prevent significant pH changes upon variation of the hydrogen ion concentration by attracting or releasing a proton. Relatively weak diprotic acids (e.g., H_2CO_3, carbonic acid) are good buffers in the human body. When carbonic acid undergoes its first dissociation reaction, it forms a proton and bicarbonate ion: $H_2CO_3 \rightarrow H^+ + HCO_3^-$. The pH of the system is due to the concentration of H^+ formed by the dissociation of H_2CO_3. Upon addition of H^+, the bicarbonate ion will become protonated so the total H^+ concentration of the medium remains about the same. Similarly, upon addition of OH-, the bicarbonate ion releases a hydrogen to form water with the OH-. This maintains the H^+ concentration and hence keeps the pH constant. These reactions are illustrated below:

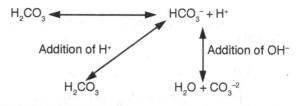

2.3   Organic Compounds

Organic compounds are complex compounds that contain carbon. They always include hydrogen. Other elements may be found in the molecules. There are four families of organic compounds with important biological functions.

2.3.1   Carbohydrates

Carbohydrate molecules consist of carbon, hydrogen, and oxygen. They have a general molecular formula of $C_n(H_2O)_n$. There are several subfamilies based on molecular size.

Monosaccharides - Monosaccharides are the building blocks of larger carbohydrate molecules. They are simple sugars. Important monosaccharides include **glucose** (blood sugar), **fructose**, and **galactose**. These three monosaccharides have the same molecular formula of $C_6H_{12}O_6$, but different structural formulas (see figure on the next page). Molecules with this relationship are called **isomers**.

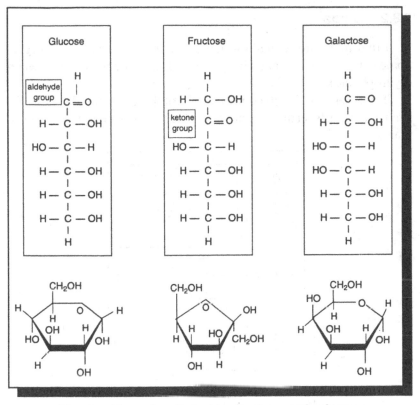

Structural formulas of glucose, fructose, and galactose

Disaccharides - Two monosaccharides bond together by a dehydration synthesis to produce a larger molecule, the disaccharide. By this
process a molecule is lost between the two smaller molecules as they
bond together, forming the larger molecule. Important disaccharides are
maltose (glucose + glucose), **sucrose** (glucose + fructose), and **lactose**
(glucose + galactose).

Polysaccharides - Many monosaccharides bond into long,
chain-like molecules called polysaccharides. **Glycogen** is the main
polysaccharide in the human body. It consists of many bonded glucose
molecules. Glycogen stores energy. Glucose is produced when glycogen
is broken down. Glucose is found in the blood. It offers an immediate
source of energy to the cells of the body.

2.3.2 Lipids

Lipid molecules contain at least carbon, hydrogen, and oxygen. Some contain nitrogen and phosphorous. Lipids are insoluble in water (hydrophobic).

Triglycerides - Triglycerides consist of three **fatty acids** bonded to a molecule of **glycerol**. They store large amounts of energy (9 calories/gram).

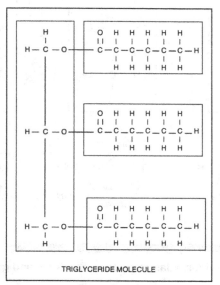

TRIGLYCERIDE MOLECULE

Structural formula of a triglyceride

Phospholipids - Phospholipids are formed when one of the fatty acids of the triglyceride is replaced by a phosphate group. They are a major component of cell membranes.

2.3.3 Proteins

All proteins contain carbon, hydrogen, oxygen, and nitrogen. Some also contain phosphorous and sulfur. The building blocks of proteins are **amino acids** (see figure on the next page). There are 20 different kinds of amino acids used by the human body. They unite by peptide bonds to form long molecules called polypeptides. Polypeptides are assembled into proteins. Proteins have four levels of structure.

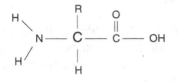

Structural formula of an amino acid

Primary Structure - The primary structure is the sequence of amino acids bonded in the polypeptide.

Secondary Structure - The secondary structure is formed by hydrogen bonds between amino acids; the polypeptide can coil into a helix or form a pleated sheet.

Tertiary Structure - The tertiary structure refers to the three-dimensional folding of the helix or pleated sheet.

Quaternary Structure - The quaternary structure refers to the spatial relationship among the polypeptides in the protein.

Proteins have the following biological functions·

Structure - They are found in hair, bones, muscles, and all cell membranes.

Regulation - Some hormones are proteins, including insulin. Insulin regulates the level of glucose in the blood.

Transport - Hemoglobin is a protein. It combines with oxygen in red blood cells as they transport oxygen.

Contraction - Actin and myosin are contractile proteins in muscle cells, producing movement.

Catalysts - All enzymes, organic catalysts, are mainly proteins.

2.3.4 Nucleic Acids

Nucleic acids are long molecules consisting of bonded subunits called **nucleotides**. A nucleotide consists of three parts: a five-carbon sugar called a deoxyribose, a nitrogenous base, and a phosphate group. The two nucleic acids that are important biologically are DNA and RNA.

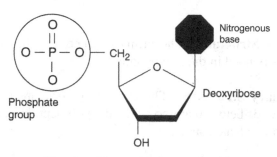

Structural formula of a nucleotide

DNA - This molecule (called deoxyribonucleic acid) consists of two long strands of bonded nucleotides. The base of each nucleotide is either adenine, cytosine, guanine, or thymine. The strands are also linked to each other through hydrogen bonding between base pairs (A-T or G-C). This ladder-like molecule is twisted into the shape of a double helix. DNA is the hereditary material of cells. It determines the development of genetic characteristics.

RNA - This molecule (called ribonucleic acid) is a single-stranded molecule of bonded nucleotides. The base of each nucleotide is either adenine, cytosine, guanine, or uracil. DNA directs the synthesis of RNA in the cell. Through this message RNA determines the synthesis of proteins.

Problem Solving Example:

Discuss some properties and functions of (a) carbohydrates, (b) lipids, (c) proteins, and (d) nucleic acids.

A (a) Carbohydrates are made up of carbon, oxygen, and hydrogen and have the general formula $C_n(H_2O)_n$. Carbohydrates can be classified as monosaccharides, disacchaides, and polysaccharides. The monosaccharides ("simple sugars") are further categorized according to the number of carbons in the molecule. Trioses contain three carbons; pentoses contain five carbons (e.g., ribose, deoxyribose); and hexoses contain six carbons (e.g., glucose, fructose, galactose). The hexoses, which exist as straight chains or rings, are important building blocks for disaccharides and the more complex carbohydrates.

Disaccharides, important in nutrition, are chemical combinations of two monosaccharides:

Lactose = glucose + galactose

Sucrose (table sugar) = glucose + fructose

Maltose = glucose + glucose

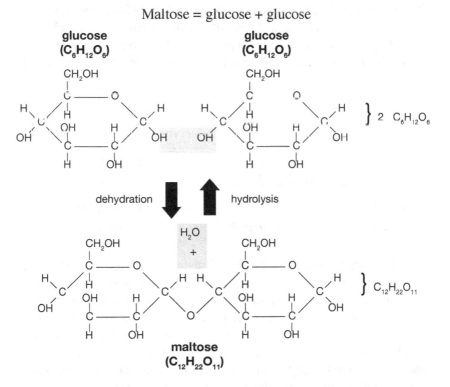

Two molecules of glucose combine to form maltose

As can be seen by the double arrows, the reverse of this reaction, hydrolysis, is also possible. Polysaccharide means "few sugars" and is arbitrarily defined as compounds that, upon hydrolysis, yield two to ten monosaccharides. Polysaccharides are complex carbohydrates made up of many monosaccharides bonded by glycosidic linkages. These long chains are formed by dehydration synthesis. They also can be broken down into monosaccharide units by hydrolysis. There are many complex polysaccharides that are of great biological significance. Their primary functions include both storage and structural properties.

(b) Lipids are also composed principally of carbon, hydrogen, and oxygen; however, they can also contain other elements, particularly phosphorus and nitrogen, and typically contain a much smaller proportion of oxygen than do carbohydrates. Lipids are insoluble in water (hydrophobic). There are many known lipids; the most common include fats and phospholipids. Fats are composed of two different types of compounds: glycerol (an alcohol) and fatty acids (organic compounds with a carboxyl group –COOH). Each molecule of fat contains one glycerol molecule and three fatty acids joined together by dehydration reactions.

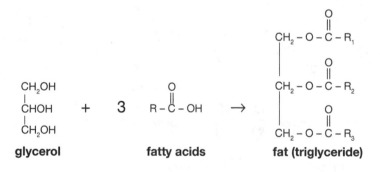

| glycerol | fatty acids | fat (triglyceride) |

There are basically two groups of fats: the saturated (those fats that have the maximum possible number of hydrogen atoms and therefore have no carbon to carbon double or triple bonds) and the unsaturated (those that have at least one carbon to carbon double or triple bond). Unsaturated fats are an important part of our diet due to their storage capabilities. Phospholipids are composed of glycerol, fatty acids, phosphoric acid, and usually a nitrogenous compound. They are important components of many cellular membranes. They are all insoluble in water, but soluble in ether.

(c) Proteins are much more complex than either carbohydrates or lipids. They are made up of the four essential elements—carbon, hydrogen, oxygen, and nitrogen—which bond together to form compounds called amino acids. Some amino acids contain sulfur. The amino acid is represented as:

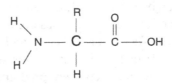

where R is a chain that can be very simple (as in the amino acid glycine where R = H) or it can be very complex (as in tryptophan where R contains two ring structures). Proteins are long and complex polymers of varying combinations of 20 amino acids that are formed by condensation reactions between the $-COO^-$ and $^-NH_3^+$ groups of the amino acid building blocks. The bonds formed by these reactions are called peptide bonds. A dipeptide is a molecule with two amino acids joined together by one peptide bond. A tripeptide refers to three linked amino acids. Oligopeptide, which includes tripeptides, is the term for a short chain of amino acids. Polypeptides are polymers of amino acids and may contain 1,000 amino acids. Finally, a protein is one or more polypeptide chains coiled or folded into complex three-dimensional configurations (primary, tertiary, or quaternary structures). Often a metal ion or organic molecule is an integral part of the protein structure. Proteins are found in every part of the cell and are an integral part in both the structure and function of living things. They play an important part in many of the chemical reactions that occur within cells because the enzymes that catalyze these reactions are proteins themselves. Proteins also function as the structural and binding materials of organisms. Hair, fingernails, muscle, cartilage, tendons, and ligaments are all structures that contain large amounts of proteins.

(d) Nucleic acids, as their name implies, are found primarily in the nucleus. There are two types of nucleic acid: deoxyribonucleic acid (DNA) and ribonucleic acid (RNA). DNA and RNA molecules are very long chains composed of repeating subunits called nucleotides. A nucleotide is composed of a five-carbon sugar (ribose in RNA; deoxyribose in DNA), a phosphate group, and any one of the following five nitrogenous bases: adenine, guanine, cytosine, thymine (only in DNA), or uracil (only in RNA). Both DNA and RNA are composed of many nucleotides linked together and are called polynucleotides or nucleic acids. In a polynucleotide, any two nucleotides are linked together by a dehydration reaction between the phosphate group of one nucleotide and the sugar group of another. The bases are attached to the sugars. Nucleic acids primarily function in heredity and govern the synthesis of many different kinds of proteins and other substances present in organisms. Chromosomes and genes are predominantly composed of DNA. Some DNA is also found in the mitochondria and the chloroplasts. Large quantities of RNA are present in the nucleoli, the cytoplasm, and the ribosomes of most cells.

Quiz: Human Body and Chemistry of Life

1. Which of the following statements is true?

   (A) DNA contains the pentose sugar ribose, while RNA contains deoxyribose.

   (B) Both DNA and RNA are double-stranded.

   (C) Both DNA and RNA contain the bases adenine and thymine.

   (D) Only RNA uses the base uracil, while only DNA contains thymine.

   (E) DNA has a pentose sugar, while RNA has a hexose.

2. Hydrogen ions are not free to lower the blood's pH because they are

   (A) removed through the action of carbonic anhydrase.

   (B) bound to water.

(C) bound to hemoglobin.

(D) removed by diffusion.

(E) bound to carbon dioxide.

3. Which of the following is the most important monosaccharide?

(A) Glucose   (D) Galactose

(B) Fructose   (E) Lactose

(C) Sucrose

4. Normally the various body fluid compartments are in osmotic equilibrium. Therefore, a net loss of solute from the extracellular fluid initially

(A) leads to hypotonicity of the extracellular fluid relative to the intracellular fluid.

(B) leads to hypotonicity of the intracellular fluid relative to the extracellular fluid.

(C) leads to hypertonicity of the extracellular fluid relative to the intracellular fluid.

(D) does not change the tonicity of the extracellular fluid or intracellular fluid.

(E) leads to isotonicity of the intracellular fluid relative to the extracellular fluid.

5. With the exception of blood cells, exchanges of water and solutes between the intracellular compartment and the plasma

(A) can occur directly.

(B) do not take place at all.

(C) occur only in highly perfused organs, such as the lungs and kidneys.

(D) can occur only indirectly, via movement through the interstitial fluid.

(E) can occur only indirectly, via movement through the intestine.

6. Amino acids with side chains that consist only of hydrocarbons are

(A) hydrophobic.   (D) hydrophilic.

(B) enantiomers.   (E) basic.

(C) zwitterions.

7. The three molecules shown below are best described as

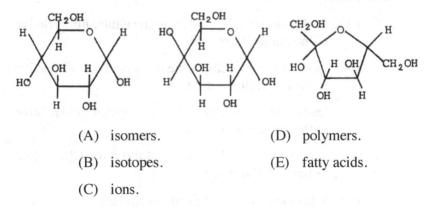

(A) isomers.   (D) polymers.

(B) isotopes.   (E) fatty acids.

(C) ions.

8. Which of the following molecules has an NH_2 group, COOH group, H group, and a variable group all attached to the same carbon?

(A) Nucleotide   (D) Fatty acid

(B) Steroid   (E) Glycerol

(C) Amino acid

9. Sodium ions function as

    (A) glucose carrier molecules.

    (B) maltose carrier molecules.

    (C) the maintainers of osmolarity.

    (D) the maintainers of tonicity.

    (E) the maintainers of the electrochemical gradient.

10. The uncharged polar side chains of several of the amino acids are most likely involved in

    (A) peptide bonds.

    (B) hydrogen bonds.

    (C) covalent bonds.

    (D) hydrophobic interactions.

    (E) disulfide bonds.

ANSWER KEY

1.	(D)	6.	(A)
2.	(C)	7.	(A)
3.	(A)	8.	(C)
4.	(A)	9.	(E)
5.	(D)	10.	(B)

CHAPTER 3

Cells

3.1   Cell Structures

The cell is the smallest unit displaying the characteristics of life. It is the unit of structure and unit of function of the human body. Cells are studied through the light microscope and electron microscope. Observations through the electron microscope reveal details of the membrane, nucleus, cytoplasm, and organelles of cell structure.

Problem Solving Example:

Q   What is a cell?

A   A cell is the fundamental organizational unit of life. One of the most important generalizations of modern biology is the cell theory. There are two components of the cell theory. It states (1) that all living things are composed of cells and (2) that all cells arise from other cells. Living things are chemical organizations of cells and capable of reproducing themselves.

There are many types of cells and just as many classifications to go with them. There are plant cells, animal cells, eukaryotic cells, procaryotic cells, and many others. Also, within each of these divisions, there are smaller subdivisions pertaining to the specific properties or functions of the cells. Cells exhibit considerable variation in properties based on different arrangements of components. Cells also vary in size, although most of them fall in the range of 1 to 100 μm.

3.1.1 Cell Membrane

The cell membrane, or plasma membrane, is the boundary of the cell. This boundary separates the outside of the cell (extracellular environment) from the inside of the cell (intracellular environment). This membrane consists of a double layer of lipid molecules. Proteins are embedded within this lipid bilayer.

The cell membrane regulates the passage of substances into and out of the cell; therefore, it is a **semipermeable** membrane. Water passes freely through the membrane. Other molecules may pass through depending on their size and charge and the ability of the membrane to recognize and transport them.

Problem Solving Example:

Describe the structure and functions of the cell membrane.

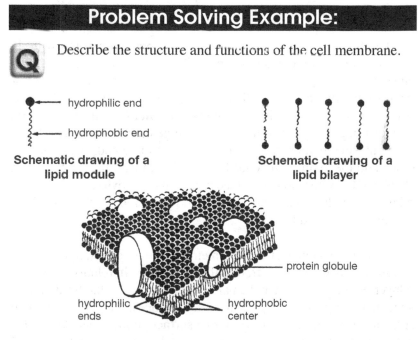

hydrophilic end

hydrophobic end

Schematic drawing of a lipid module

Schematic drawing of a lipid bilayer

protein globule

hydrophilic ends

hydrophobic center

Model of the unit membrane

A   Each cell is surrounded by a selective membrane, a complex elastic covering that separates the cell protoplasm from the external environment. The structure of this covering, called the cell, or plasma, membrane, has been under major investigation for many years. Studies of membrane permeability, electron microscopy, and biochemical analysis have enabled biologists to better understand the structure and composition of the plasma membrane. The cell membrane contains about 40 percent lipid and 60 percent protein by weight, with considerable variation from cell type to cell type. The different types and amounts of lipids and proteins present determine to a great extent the characteristics of different membranes. As seen in electron micrographs, all membranes appear to have a similar fundamental structure. The cell membrane is revealed by electron microscopy to resemble a railroad track cross-section—two dark lines bordering a central lighter line. The membranes of cellular organelles also display this characteristic. The two dark lines suggested a correspondence to two layers of protein and the light middle layer to lipid. It was soon revealed that the lipid actually exists in two layers.

The lipid molecules of the plasma membrane are polar, with the two ends of each molecule having different electric properties. One end is hydrophobic (literally "fear of water"), which means it tends to be insoluble in water. The other end is hydrophilic (literally "love of water"), which means it has an affinity for water (see the figure on the previous page). The lipid molecules arrange themselves in two layers in the plasma membrane so that the hydrophobic ends are near each other, and the hydrophilic ends face outside toward the water and are stabilized by water molecules (see figure on the previous page). In this bilayer, individual lipid molecules can move laterally so that the bilayer is actually fluid and flexible.

Protein molecules of the cell membrane may be arranged in various sites by being embedded to different degrees in relationship to the bilayer. Some of them may be partially embedded in the lipid bilayer; some may be present only on the outer surfaces; and still others may span the entire lipid bilayer from one surface to the other. The different arrangements of proteins are determined by the different structural, conformational, and electrical characteristics of various membrane proteins. Like the lipid bilayer, the protein molecules tend to orient themselves in the most stable way possible. The proteins are usually folded naturally into a globular form, which enables them to move laterally within the plane of the membrane at different rates. Certain proteins can actually move across the membrane. Thus, membrane proteins are not static but dynamic.

The functions of the cell membrane are highly specific and directly related to its structure, which is, in turn, dependent on the specific types and amounts of proteins and lipids present. The discriminating permeability of the membrane is its primary function. It allows certain substances to enter or leave the cell and prevents other substances from crossing it. Whether or not a molecule can cross a membrane depends on its size after hydration, electric charge, shape, chemical properties, and its relative solubility in lipid as compared to that in water. This selective permeability of the cell membrane gives the cell the ability to keep its interior environment both chemically and physically different from the exterior environment.

The cell membrane is also found to be particularly important in cell adherence. Because of the specificity of protein molecules on the membrane surface, cells can recognize each other and bind together through some interaction of their surface proteins. Surface proteins are believed to provide communication and linkage between cells in division so that cells divide in an organized plane, rather than in random directions, which gives rise to an amorphous mass of cells (e.g., cancer). Surface proteins of the cell membrane also recognize foreign substances; they can bind with the foreign substance and inactivate it. Membrane proteins are further suggested to interact with hormones or convey hormonal messages to the nucleus so that a physiological change can be effected. The cell membrane also is involved in the conduction of impulse in nerve cells. The axon of nerve cells transmits impulses by a temporary redistribution of ions inside and outside the cell, with a subsequent change in the distribution of charges on the two surfaces of the membrane.

3.1.2 Nucleus

The nucleus is defined by a double membrane, the **nuclear envelope**. There are pores in this envelope. The nucleus controls the characteristics and functions of the cell. **Chromatin**, a mass of thread-like material, is found in the nucleus. The chromatin condenses into rod-like structures called **chromosomes** during cell division. Each chromosome carries a series of genes, the units of heredity. The genes are composed of DNA.

The **nucleolus** is an oval body found inside the nucleus. It consists of RNA and protein. Nucleoli are made by the chromosomes and participate in protein synthesis.

Problem Solving Example:

Q What are the functions of the nucleus? What is the evidence that indicates the role of the nucleus in cell metabolism and heredity?

A If the cell is thought of as a miniature chemical plant designed to carry out all the processes of life, then the nucleus can be compared to a central computer that controls a network of sophisticated and highly complicated biochemical machinery. This is because the nucleus contains the chromosomes, which bear the genes, the ultimate regulators of life.

The genes comprise a library of programs stored in the nucleus: programs that specify the precise nature of each protein synthesized by the cell. The nucleus monitors changing conditions both inside the cell and in the external environment and responds to input of information by either activating or inhibiting the appropriate genetic programs.

Control of protein synthesis is the key to controlling the activities and responses of the cell since a tremendous array of important biological and biochemical processes are regulated by enzymatic proteins. By switching particular genes on and off, the cell controls not only the kinds of enzymes that it produces, but also the amounts. Both qualitative and quantitative control of enzyme synthesis are crucial to the proper functioning of the cell and the whole organism.

The nucleus is of central importance also in the transmission of hereditary information. The nucleus carries the information for all the characteristics of the cell. This information is found in the chromosomes, which consist of protein and DNA. When the cell divides, the nuclear information is transmitted in an orderly fashion to the daughter cells by replication of the chromosomes and division of the nucleus. Thus, in this type of division, the daughter cells each possess a single complement of genetic information identical to that of the mother cell.

3.1.3 Cytoplasm

The cytoplasm is the material found between the nucleus and cell membrane. It consists of water and different organic molecules. Various organelles are embedded in the cytoplasm.

Problem Solving Example:

Describe the makeup of cytoplasm.

The cytoplasm of a living cell is a watery medium separated from the external environment by the plasma membrane. The cytoplasm resembles a loose gel that is somewhat denser than pure water. In order to move from one part of a cell to another, materials have to move through this relatively dense gel.

3.1.4 Organelles

The organelles are the distinct bodies contained within the cytoplasm. Each organelle has a distinctive structure and function.

Centriole - The centriole is a short cylinder near the nuclear envelope. Normally there are two centrioles at right angles to each other. They coordinate the events of cell division.

Problem Solving Example:

Q Describe the structure of a centriole. What function does it serve?

A Centrioles are small bodies located just outside the nucleus of the cell in a specialized region of cytoplasm that has been known to play a role in cell division. Centrioles usually occur as a pair in each cell and are oriented at right angles to each other. Each centriole of the pair is composed of nine groups of tubules arranged longitudinally in a ring to form a hollow cylinder. Each group is a triplet composed of three closely associated tubular elements called microtubules (see figures). The space immediately surrounding a pair of centrioles is called the centrosome. The centrosome appears to be clear or empty under the spectroscope.

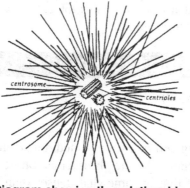

centrosome

centrioles

**Diagram showing the relationship of
the centrioles and centrosome**

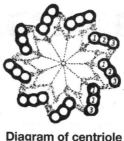

**Diagram of centriole
structure**

The centrioles seem to play some part in directing the orderly distribution of genetic material during cell division. At the beginning of cell division, the centrioles replicate and the two pairs of centrioles that result move to opposite poles of the dividing cell. Under the electron microscope, each pair is seen to send out spindle fibers, structures involved in separating and moving chromosomes to the opposite ends of the cell. This observation leads to the hypothesis that centrioles are needed in the formation of the spindle fibers; however, cells capable of spindle formation without centrioles seem to refute this hypothesis.

Endoplasmic Reticulum (ER) - The ER is a membranous series of tubular channels. It is contiguous within the nuclear envelope. It provides a passageway for the transport of substances. The rough ER is covered with ribosomes. The smooth ER is not covered with ribosomes.

Problem Solving Example:

 Explain the importance and structure of the endoplasmic reticulum in the cell.

The endoplasmic reticulum is responsible for transporting certain molecules to specific areas within the cytoplasm. Lipids and proteins are synthesized and distributed by this system. The endoplasmic reticulum is more than a passive channel for intracellular transport. It contains a variety of enzymes playing important roles in metabolic processes.

The structure of the endoplasmic reticulum is a complex of membranes that traverses the cytoplasm. The membranes form interconnecting channels that take the form of flattened sacs and tubes. When the endoplasmic reticulum has ribosomes attached to its surface, we refer to it as rough endoplasmic reticulum, and when there are no ribosomes attached, it is called smooth endoplasmic reticulum. The rough endoplasmic reticulum functions in transport of cellular products; the role of the smooth endoplasmic reticulum is less well known, but is believed to be involved in lipid synthesis (thus the predominance of smooth endoplasmic reticulum in hepatocytes of the liver).

In most cells, the endoplasmic reticulum is continuous and interconnected at some points with the nuclear membrane and, sometimes, with the plasma membrane. This may indicate a pathway by which materials synthesized in the nucleus are transported to the cytoplasm. In cells actively engaged in protein synthesis and secretion (such as acinar cells of the pancreas), rough endoplasmic reticulum is abundant. By a well-regulated and organized process, protein or polypeptide chains are synthesized on the ribosomes. These products are then transported by the endoplasmic reticulum to other sites of the cell where they are needed. If they are secretory products, they have to be packaged for release. They are carried by the endoplasmic reticulum to the Golgi apparatus, another organelle system. Some terminal portions of the endoplasmic reticulum containing protein molecules bud off from the membranes of the reticulum complex and move to the Golgi apparatus in the form of membrane-bound vesicles. In the Golgi apparatus, the protein molecules are concentrated, chemically modified, and packaged so that they can be released to the outside by exocytosis. This process is necessary because some proteins may be digestive enzymes, which may degrade the cytoplasm and lyse the cell if direct contact is made.

Ribosome - The ribosomes are small particles consisting of RNA. They are the site of protein synthesis.

Problem Solving Example:

 What is the function and location of ribosomes?

The small spherical bodies that we see studding the endoplasmic reticulum—more accurately, the rough endoplasmic reticulum— are the ribosomes. The rough endoplasmic reticulum owes its rough appearance to the presence of ribosomes. The smooth endoplasmic reticulum appears smooth because it lacks ribosomes. Ribosomes consist of two parts, a large subunit and a small subunit. Both the large and small subunits are made of proteins and RNA. However, the two subunits differ both in the number and in the type of proteins and RNA they contain. The large subunit contains larger and more varied RNA molecules than the small subunit. It also has more protein molecules than the smaller one. An interesting point to note is that when we put together all the chemical components of a ribosome, under favorable conditions, these parts will rearrange themselves and come together, without direction from preexisting ribosomes, to form a functional assembly. This ability to self-assemble may provide us with a clue to the origin of living things.

Ribosomes are the sites of protein synthesis in the cell. Messenger RNA (mRNA), which carries genetic information from the nucleus,

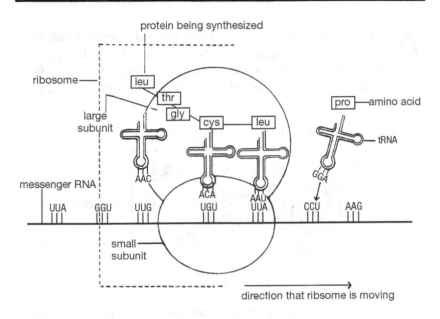

protein being synthesized

ribosome

large subunit

messenger RNA

small subunit

direction that ribosome is moving

The role of the ribosome in protein synthesis

associates with the small ribosomal subunit first and then binds to the large subunit as a prelude to protein synthesis. This association of mRNA to ribosomes holds the components of the complex system of protein synthesis together in a specific manner for greater efficiency than if they were dispersed freely in the cytoplasm. The mRNA then pairs with complementary molecules of transfer RNA (tRNA), each carrying a specific amino acid. The linking up of tRNA molecules into a chain complementary to mRNA brings together amino acids that bind with each other to form a highly specific protein molecule. Thus, ribosomes are the sites where proteins are synthesized under genetic control.

Golgi Apparatus - This organelle is a series of flattened vacuoles. They package, store, and modify products that will be secreted from the cell.

Problem Solving Example:

How is the Golgi apparatus related to the endoplasmic reticulum in function?

A The Golgi apparatus is composed of flat, membranous sacs, or cisternae, arranged in stacks. These stacks have two poles — the *cis* face, which receives materials for processing, and the *trans* face, through which substances are released for transport to other parts of the cell.

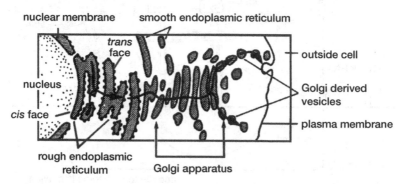

nuclear membrane   smooth endoplasmic reticulum

trans face

nucleus

cis face

outside cell

Golgi derived vesicles

plasma membrane

rough endoplasmic reticulum   Golgi apparatus

Schematic representation of the secretion of a protein in a typical animal cell. The solid arrow represents the probable route of secreted proteins.

Proteins are synthesized on the rough endoplasmic reticulum. These proteins are transferred to the Golgi apparatus by transport vesicles, which fuse with the *cis* face of the Golgi membrane. In the Golgi apparatus, the protein is concentrated by removal of water. In addition, chemical modifications of the protein, such as glycosylation (addition of sugar) occur. The modified protein is released from the *trans* face through vesicles that separate from the Golgi and travel to other parts of the cell.

Mitochondrion - Mitochondria are the powerhouses of the cell. Each one has a double membrane, which is the site of chemical reactions that extract energy from nutrient molecules.

Problem Solving Example:

Q Why are the mitochondria referred to as the "powerhouses of the cell"?

A Mitochondria are membrane-bounded organelles concerned principally with the generation of energy to support the various forms of chemical and mechanical work carried out by the cell. Mitochondria are distributed throughout the cell because all parts of it require energy. Mitochondria tend to be most numerous in regions of the cell that consume large amounts of energy and more abundant in cells that require a great deal of energy (e.g., muscle and sperm cells).

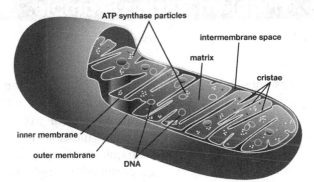

Diagram showing the internal structures of a mitochondrion through a cutaway view

Mitochondria are enclosed by two membranes. The outer one is a continuous delimiting membrane. The inner membrane is thrown into many folds that extend into the interior of the mitochondrion. These folds are called cristae. Enclosed by the inner membrane is the ground substance termed the matrix (see accompanying diagram). Many enzymes involved in the Krebs cycle are found in the matrix. Enzymes involved in the generation of ATP (adenosine triphosphate) by the oxidation of $NaDH_2$ or the electron transport reactions are tightly bound to the inner mitochondrial membrane. The enzymes for the specific pathways are arranged in sequential order so that the products of one reaction do not have to travel far before they are likely to encounter the enzymes catalyzing the next reaction. This promotes a highly efficient energy production.

The reactions that occur in the mitochondria are all related in that they result in the production of ATP, which is the common currency of energy conversion in the cell. Some ATP is produced by reactions that occur in the cytoplasm, but about 95 percent of all ATP produced in the cell is in the mitochondria. For this reason the mitochondria are commonly referred to as the powerhouses of the cell.

Lysosome - Lysosomes are membrane-enclosed organelles containing digestive enzymes. The release of these enzymes can break down substances.

Problem Solving Example:

Why do cells contain lysosomes?

Lysosomes are membrane-bounded bodies in the cell. All lysosomes function in, directly or indirectly, intracellular digestion. The material to be digested may be of extracellular or intracellular origin. Lysosomes contain enzymes known collectively as acid hydrolases. These enzymes can quickly dissolve all the major molecules that constitute the cell and presumably would do so if they were not confined in structures surrounded by membranes.

One function of lysosomes is to accomplish the self-destruction of injured cells or cells that have outlived their usefulness. Lysosomes also destroy certain organelles that are no longer useful. Lysosomes are, in addition, involved in the digestion of materials taken into the cell in membranous vesicles. Lysosomes fuse with the membrane of the vesicle so that their hydrolytic enzymes are discharged into the vesicle and ultimately digest the material. Lysosomes play a part in the breakdown of normal cellular waste products and in the turnover of cellular constituents.

Vacuole - Various membrane-bound vacuoles can store water, nutrients, or waste products in the cell.

Peroxisome - This membrane-bound organelle contains enzymes for oxidation reactions in the cell.

Problem Solving Example:

Q What are peroxisomes and how do they function in a cell?

A Peroxisomes are similar to lysosomes but differ in two ways. Lysosomes are a product of the Golgi apparatus, whereas peroxisomes are formed by budding off from the endoplasmic reticulum. Second, peroxisomes contain enzymes for oxidation rather than hydrolases. Peroxisome enzymes are capable of combining with oxygen and hydrogen, forming hydrogen peroxide (H_2O_2), a highly oxidizing substance. Hydrogen peroxide in association with catalase, another oxidizing enzyme present in peroxisomes, prevents the cell from being poisoned by an otherwise toxic substance. An example of this reaction occurs in the liver when it detoxifies alcohol that is consumed. Another specific function of hydrogen peroxide–catalase-oxidizing reactions is to break down fatty acids into acetyl-CoA, which is used for energy by the cell.

Cytoskeleton - Several kinds of proteins in the cytoplasm form the cytoskeleton. Microfilaments are long, thin fibers. Microtubules are thin cylinders. They maintain cell shape and influence cell movement.

Problem Solving Example:

Q Microtubules and microfilaments both appear to be involved in intracellular motion and in the cytoskeleton. How do the two organelles differ in structure and function, and how are they similar?

A Microtubules are thin, hollow cylinders, approximately 200 to 300 Angstroms in diameter. Microfilaments are not hollow and are 50 to 80 Angstroms in diameter. Both microtubules and microfilaments are composed of proteins. The protein of microtubules is generally termed tubulin. Tubule proteins can be made to assemble into microtubules in a test tube, if the proper reagents are present. Some of the narrower microfilaments have been shown to be composed of proteins similar to actin. Actin is a protein involved in muscle cell contraction. The composition of thicker microfilaments has not been completely determined.

Microtubules are often distributed in cells in arrangements that suggest their role in maintaining cell shape (a "cytoskeletal" role). For example, microtubules are arranged longitudinally within the elongated processes of nerve cells (axons) and the cytoplasmic extensions (pseudopods) of certain protozoa. Microtubules are arranged in a circular band in the disc-shaped fish red blood cells. Microfilaments may also play a structural role. They are often associated with some specialized region of the cell membrane, such as the absorptive cell membrane of the intestinal cells, or the portions of the cell membrane that serve to anchor adjacent cells together so that they can communicate.

Microtubules are components of cilia and flagella and participate in the rapid movements of these structures. Microtubules are involved in directional movement within the cell during cell division and are involved in certain types of oriented rapid intracellular movement. Microfilaments seem to be involved in many different types of cytoplasmic movement. Close associations between microfilaments and membrane bound organelles suggest that microfilaments assist in intracellular transport and exchange of materials.

Cilium - The cilium is a short, hair-like projection from the cell membrane. The coordinated beating of many cilia produces organized movement.

Flagellum - A flagellum is a long, whip-like organelle extending from the cell membrane. Its action produces movement.

Problem Solving Example:

 Explain the structural and functional aspects of cilia and flagella.

 Some cells have one or more hair-like or whip-like protuberances projecting from their surfaces. If there are only one or two of these appendages and they are relatively long in proportion to the size of the cell, they are called flagella. If there are many that are short, they are called cilia. Actually, the basic structure of flagella and cilia is the same. They resemble centrioles in having nine sets of microtubules arranged in a cylinder. But unlike centrioles, each set is a doublet rather than a triplet of microtubules, and two singlets are present in the center of the cylinder. At the base of the cylinders of cilia and flagella, within the main portion of the cell, is a basal body. The basal body is essential to the functioning of the cilia and flagella. From the basal body, fibers project into the cytoplasm, possibly to anchor the basal body to the cell.

Both cilia and flagella usually function either by moving the cell or by moving liquids or small particles across the surface of the cell. Flagella move with an undulating snake-like motion. Cilia beat in co-ordinated waves. Both move by the contraction of the tubular proteins contained within them.

3.2 Cell Transport

Molecules are transported into and out of the cell. They are also transported between regions within the cell. Transport processes include diffusion, osmosis, active transport, filtration, endocytosis, and exocytosis.

Diffusion - Diffusion is the movement of molecules from a region of higher concentration to a region of lower concentration. Oxygen diffuses from the blood into the cells of the body. Diffusion is a passive process, as it does not require an energy output from the cell.

Problem Solving Example:

 Why is the phenomenon of diffusion important to movement of materials in living cells?

 In a living cell, chemical reactions are constantly taking place to produce the energy or organic compounds needed to main-tain life. The reacting materials of chemical reactions must be supplied continuously to the actively metabolizing cell and the products distributed to other parts of the cell where they are needed or where they are lower in concentration. This is extremely important because if the reactants are not supplied, the reaction ceases. If the products are not distributed but instead accumulate near the site of reaction, LeChatelier's Principle of chemical reactions operates to drive the reversible reaction backward, diminishing the concentration of the products. Thus, in order to maintain a chemical reaction, the reactants must be continuously supplied and the products must move through the cell medium to other sites. Diffusion is how these processes occur.

When a certain chemical reaction is operating in the cell, some reacting substance will be used. The concentration of this substance is necessarily lower in regions closer to the site of reaction than regions farther away from it. Under this condition, a concentration gradient is established. The concentration gradient causes the movement of molecules of this substance from a region of higher concentration to a region of lower concentration, or the reaction site. This movement is called diffusion. Thus, by diffusion, molecules tend to move to regions in the cell where they are being consumed. The products of the reaction travel away from the reaction site also by this process of diffusion. At the reaction site, the concentration of the products is highest; hence, the products tend to move away from this region to ones where they are lower in concentration. The removal of products signals the reaction to continue. When the product concentration gets too high, the reaction is inhibited by a built-in feedback mechanism.

Thus, diffusion explains how movement of chemical substances occurs into or out of the cell and within the cell. For example, oxygen molecules are directed by a concentration gradient to enter the cell and move toward the mitochondria. This is because oxygen concentration is necessarily the lowest in the mitochondria, where oxidation reactions continually consume oxygen. Carbon dioxide is produced when an acetyl unit is completely oxidized in the citric acid cycle. The CO_2 will then travel away from the mitochondria, where it is produced, to other parts of the cell, or out of the cell into the bloodstream, where it is lower in concentration.

Osmosis - Osmosis is the diffusion of water through a semipermeable membrane. A cell can lose water to a **hypertonic** medium by osmosis. This medium has a higher concentration of solute molecules; therefore, its concentration of water is less and water will diffuse toward it. A cell will gain water from a **hypotonic** medium. This medium has a lower concentration of solute molecules; therefore, its concentration of water is greater, and water will leave it to enter the cell.

Normally, the extracellular environment is **isotonic**. This means that the solute concentrations are equal. In this case, the cell does not lose or gain water.

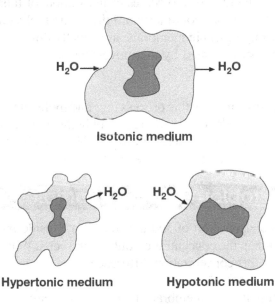

Isotonic medium

Hypertonic medium   Hypotonic medium

Osmotic effects on a cell in hypertonic, hypotonic, and isotonic environments

Problem Solving Example:

Q How does water move by osmosis?

A Most cells are surrounded by a semipermeable membrane that is permeable to water but not to all solute particles or molecules. Osmosis is the passage of water across a semipermeable membrane. Osmosis is regulated by the concentration of solute molecules. This process is regulated by the concentration of nondiffusible particles on either side of the semipermeable membrane. Water moving from the side of the membrane that has the lesser number of molecules to the side with the greater number of molecules is an example of this principle. This movement of water continues until the solute molecules on both sides of the semipermeable membrane are equally diluted or until the hydrostatic pressure created by the movement of water opposes this movement.

Active Transport - By this process ions and molecules move from a region of lower concentration to a region of higher concentration. The cell must expend energy for active transport. Nerve cells, for example, actively transport sodium ions to the extracellular environment.

Problem Solving Example:

Q The concentration of sodium ions (Na⁺) inside most cells is lower than the concentration outside the cells. What process is responsible for this concentration difference?

A Because the cell membrane is somewhat permeable to sodium ions, simple diffusion would result in a net movement of sodium ions into the cell, until the concentrations on the two sides of the membrane became equal. Sodium actually does diffuse into the cell rather freely, but as fast as it does so, the cell actively pumps it out again, against the concentration gradient.

The mechanism by which the cell pumps the sodium ions out is called active transport. Active transport requires the expenditure of energy for the work done by the cell in moving molecules against a concentration gradient. Active transport enables a cell to maintain a lower concentration of sodium inside the cell, and also enables a cell to accumulate certain nutrients inside the cell at concentrations much higher than the extracellular concentrations.

The exact mechanism of active transport is not known. It has been proposed that a carrier molecule is involved, which reacts chemically with the molecule that is to be actively transported. This forms a compound that is soluble in the lipid portion of the membrane, and the carrier compound then moves through the membrane against the concentration gradient to the other side. The transported molecule is then released, and the carrier molecule diffuses back to the other side of the membrane, where it picks up another molecule. This process requires energy, since work must be done in transporting the molecule against a diffusion gradient. The energy is supplied in the form of ATP.

The carrier molecules are thought to be integral proteins, proteins that span the cell membrane. These proteins are specific for the molecules they transport.

Filtration - Molecules pass through membranes by physical force during filtration. For example, blood pressure forces substances across the thin walls of capillaries by filtration. By this process, water and other molecules leave the circulation to serve the cells of the body.

Endocytosis - Through endocytosis the cell actively encloses an extracellular particle, forming a membrane-bound vesicle in the cell. If the particle is solid, this is called phagocytosis. If it is a liquid, it is called pinocytosis. Leukocytes (white blood cells) protect the body by phagocytosis.

Exocytosis - This is the reverse of endocytosis. The cell discharges membrane-bound substances that were intracellular.

Problem Solving Example:

 Distinguish between the terms "endocytosis" and "exocytosis."

 The transport of macromolecules through the plasma membrane is accomplished by the processes of endocytosis and exocytosis. In exocytosis, an intracellular vesicle is transported to the plasma membrane, where it fuses with the plasma membrane. The fusion process releases the contents of the vesicle to the extracellular space. Endocytosis is essentially the reverse of this process.

3.3 Cell Reproduction

There are two types of cell reproduction that occur in the human body. Body cells reproduce by mitosis. This type of cell division is necessary for growth and tissue repair. Meiosis is the other kind of cell division. Through meiosis, sex cells are produced.

3.3.1 Mitosis

During mitosis, one parent cell divides to produce two daughter cells. Each parent cell in the human body normally has 46 chromosomes. By mitosis each daughter cell produced will receive the same number and kinds of chromosomes as the original parent cell. The identity of the genes on each chromosome will also be the same.

Mitosis is part of the entire life span of the cell, also called the cell cycle. This entire cycle consists of the following stages:

Interphase - The nuclear envelope of the cell is intact and the nucleolus is visible. The chromosomes are not visible, appearing as chromatin. Interphase makes up the majority of the cell cycle. The cell is carrying out its normal functions: synthesizing, transporting, and storing substances. It is also preparing for cell division. Duplication of the chromosomes is one of the important steps of preparation.

Prophase - This is the first active stage of mitosis. The nuclear envelope and nucleolus disappear. The chromosomes become distinct, appearing double-stranded. The duplicates of each chromosome are called **chromatids**. The chromatids are attached at a region called the **centromere**. The centrioles migrate to opposite poles of the cell, organizing a mitotic spindle. Near the end of prophase, the chromosomes migrate toward the spindle.

Metaphase - The chromosomes line up and attach along the center of the mitotic spindle. This central region is the equator. Each double-stranded chromosome attaches to a different spindle fiber by its centromere.

Anaphase - The centromere of each chromosome splits, separating the duplicates (chromatids) of each chromosome. The duplicates of each chromosome are pulled toward opposite ends of the cell by the contraction of the spindle fibers. **Cytokinesis**, cytoplasmic division, begins.

Telophase - Cytokinesis is complete as the parent cell is pinched into two separate daughter cells. Each daughter cell contains one copy of each chromosome; therefore, the daughter cells are genetically identical. Most of the other events of telophase are the reverse of prophase. For example, the nuclear envelope and nucleolus reappear and the chromosomes disappear.

Problem Solving Example:

Outline briefly the events occurring in each stage of mitosis. Illustrate your discussion with diagrams if necessary.

Mitosis refers to the process by which a cell divides to form two daughter cells, each with exactly the same number and kind of chromosomes as the parent cell. In a strict sense, mitosis refers to the division of nuclear material (karyokinesis). Cytokinesis is the term used to refer to the division of the cytoplasm. Although each cell division is a continuous process, in order for it to be studied, it can be artificially divided into a number of stages. We will describe each stage separately, beginning with interphase.

1. Interphase: This phase is called the resting stage. However, the cell is "resting" only with respect to the visible events of division in later phases. During this phase, the nucleus is metabolically very active, and chromosomal duplication is occurring. During interphase, the chromosomes appear as vague, dispersed thread-like structures, and are referred to as chromatin material.

2. Prophase: Prophase begins when the chromatin threads begin to condense and appear as a tangled mass of threads within the nucleus. Each prophase chromosome is composed of two identical members resulting from duplication in interphase. Each member of the pair is called a chromatid. The two chromatids are held together at a dark, constricted area called the centromere. At this point the centromere is a single structure.

The above events occur in the nucleus of the cell. In the cytoplasm, the centriole (a cytoplasmic structure involved in division) divides and the two daughter centrioles migrate to opposite sides of the cell. From each centriole there extends a cluster of ray-like filaments called an aster. Between the separating centrioles, a mitotic spindle forms, composed of protein fibrils with contractile properties. In late prophase the chromosomes are fully contracted and appear as short, rod-like bodies. At this point individual chromosomes can be distinguished by their characteristic shapes and sizes. They then begin to migrate and line up along the equatorial plane of the spindle. Each doubled chromosome appears to be attached to the spindle at its centromere. The nucleolus (spherical body within the nucleus where RNA synthesis is believed to occur) has been undergoing dissolution during prophase. In addition, the nuclear envelope breaks down, and its disintegration marks the end of prophase.

3. Metaphase: When the chromosomes have all lined up and attached along the equator, the dividing cell is in metaphase. At this time, the centromere divides and the chromatids become completely separate daughter chromosomes. The division of the centromeres occurs simultaneously in all the chromosomes.

4. Anaphase: The beginning of anaphase is marked by the movement of the separated chromatids (or daughter chromosomes) to opposite poles of the cell. It is thought that the chromosomes are pulled as a result of contraction of the spindle fibers in the presence of ATP. The chromosomes moving toward the poles usually assume a V shape, with the centromere at the apex pointing toward the pole.

5. Telophase: When the chromosomes reach the poles, telophase begins. The chromosomes relax, elongate, and return to the resting condition

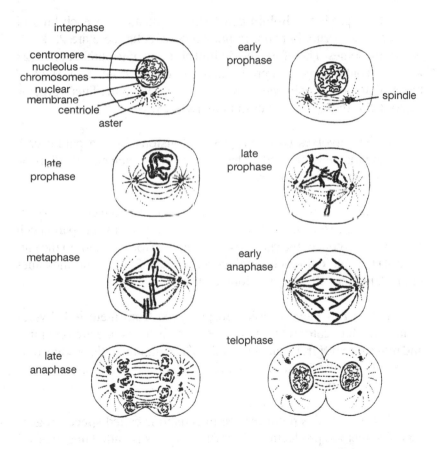

The stages of mitosis in a cell with a diploid number of 4 (2n=4)

in which only chromatin threads are visible. A nuclear membrane forms around each new daughter nucleus. This completes karyokinesis, and cytokinesis follows.

The cytoplasmic division of cells is accomplished by the formation of a furrow in the equatorial plane. The furrow gradually deepens and separates the cytoplasm into daughter cells, each with a nucleus.

3.3.2 Meiosis

Mitosis produces **diploid** cells. Diploid means that each kind of chromosome occurs in pairs. In human body cells there are 23 kinds of chromosomes. Therefore, the diploid chromosome number is 46 (23 × 2). By contrast, meiosis produces **haploid** cells (gametes). Haploid means that there is only one copy of each chromosome. Therefore, the haploid chromosome number in humans is 23.

Meiosis involves two consecutive divisions from a parent cell, producing four daughter cells. The main events of each meiotic division (meiosis I and meiosis II) are:

Meiosis I - After each chromosome duplicates, the chromosomes of each pair are separated into different daughter cells as the parent cell divides. This reduces the chromosome number from diploid (in the parent cell) to haploid (in each daughter cell). Each of the 23 chromosomes in the daughter cells remains double-stranded.

Meiosis II - Each haploid cell produced from meiosis I divides again. The duplicates (chromatids) of each chromosome are separated and move into different daughter cells. The daughter cells produced by meiosis II are also haploid. However, each of the 23 chromosomes is now single-stranded.

Meiosis in males produces sperm cells. It is called **spermatogenesis**. The meiotic production of female sex cells is called **oogenesis**.

Problem Solving Example:

Q Outline briefly the events occurring in each stage of meiosis. Illustrate your discussion with diagrams if necessary.

A Meiosis is the process by which diploid cells (having two sets of chromosomes) produce haploid gametes (having only one

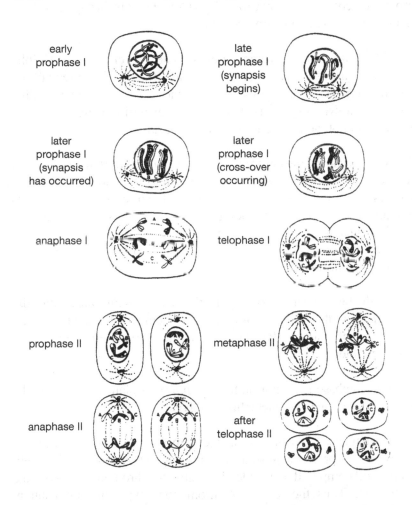

early prophase I

late prophase I (synapsis begins)

later prophase I (synapsis has occurred)

later prophase I (cross-over occurring)

anaphase I

telophase I

prophase II

metaphase II

anaphase II

after telophase II

The stages of meiosis in a cell with a diploid number of 6

set of chromosomes). When two gametes fuse in fertilization, the zygote formed will thus have the full diploid chromosomal complement.

Meiosis consists of two cell divisions, the first (meiosis I) called reduction division and the second (meiosis II) a mitotic type division.

1. Interphase I: This phase is similar to mitotic interphase. The cell appears inactive in reference to cell division, but it is during interphase that chromosome duplication occurs.

2. Prophase I: The chromosomes become thicker and more visible. While they are still long, thin threads, an attractive force (as yet not identified) causes homologous chromosomes to come together in pairs, a process known as synapsis. This is the stage during which crossover between homologous chromosomes will occur.

After synapsis, the chromosomes continue to shorten and thicken; their double nature becomes visible so that each homologous pair appears as a bundle of four chromatids called a tetrad. Each tetrad is composed of two double homologous chromosomes. The number of tetrads is thus equal to the haploid number. The centromeres of homologous chromosomes are connected, and there are thus two centromeres for the four chromatids.

While these events are occurring, the centrioles migrate to opposite poles, the spindle begins to form between them, and the nucleolus and nuclear membrane dissolve. The tetrads move to the equatorial plane of the spindle.

3. Metaphase I: Migration to the equatorial plane occurs, and the nuclear membrane and nucleolus dissolve.

4. Anaphase I: At this point, the homologous chromosomes that have paired in prophase separate and move to opposite poles of the cell. Each is still composed of two identical daughter chromatids joined at the centromere. Thus, the number of chromosome types in each resultant cell is reduced to the haploid number.

5. Telophase I: Cytoplasmic division occurs as in mitosis. Meiosis I concludes and meiosis II begins. There is no definable interphase between the two series of divisions. The chromosomes do not separate or duplicate, nor do they form chromatin threads.

6. Prophase II: The centrioles that had migrated to each pole of the parental cell, now incorporated in each haploid daughter cell, divide, and a new spindle forms in each cell. The chromosomes move to the equator.

7. Metaphase II: The chromosomes line up at the equator of the new spindle, which is at right angles to the old spindle.

8. Anaphase II: The centromeres divide, and the daughter chromatids, now chromosomes, separate and move to opposite poles.

9. Telophase II: Cytoplasmic division occurs. The chromosomes gradually return to the dispersed form, and a nuclear membrane forms.

The two meiotic divisions yield four cells, each carrying only one member of each homologous pair of chromosomes. These cells are for this reason called haploid cells.

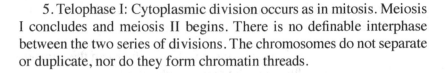

Quiz: Cells

1.   Mitosis functions in many organism life cycle events EXCEPT

    (A)   body cell replacement.

    (B)   development.

    (C)   gametogenesis.

    (D)   growth.

    (E)   wound healing.

2. All of the following statements about the cell membrane are true EXCEPT

    (A) it functions as a selective barrier between the intracellular fluid and the extracellular fluid.

    (B) the proteins within it are classified as intrinsic (integral) or extrinsic (peripheral).

    (C) the major lipid within it is cholesterol.

    (D) the fluid-mosaic model describes the fluidity and mobility of the membrane.

    (E) the phospholipids within are amphipathic—that is, they each contain polar and nonpolar regions.

3. Which of the following statements best describes transport across cell membranes?

    (A) Those transport proteins involved in active transport maintain a permanently fixed asymmetry with respect to the two sides of the membranes; this maintains the directional sense of the transport.

    (B) All active transport processes are coupled to the hydrolysis of phosphate bonds.

    (C) The flow of protons plays a role in prokaryotic transport processes analogous to that of Na^+ ions in eukaryotes.

    (D) Mediated transport may be differentiated experimentally from nonmediated transport by the presence or absence of changes in the direction of transport if the concentration gradient is reversed.

    (E) Active transport may be differentiated from passive transport because mediated diffusion by saturation affects the initial velocity of transport.

4.   Many single cells have evolved the following method for excreting cellular wastes: A vacuole containing material to be expelled travels to the cell membrane and fuses with it. After this fusion has been completed, the site of contact opens up and the contents of the vacuole are jettisoned out of the cell. This process is known as

   (A)   endocytosis.

   (B)   phagocytosis.

   (C)   pinocytosis.

   (D)   exocytosis.

   (E)   None of the above.

5.   Which of the following statements defines meiosis or the purpose of meiosis?

   (A)   The number of chromosomes in the diploid nucleus is reduced by half.

   (B)   The fusion of two haploid nuclei forms a diploid nucleus.

   (C)   The process by which four haploid cells or nuclei are transformed into a diploid cell

   (D)   The separation of chromosomes.

   (E)   The fusion of chromosomes.

6.   Facilitated diffusion

   (A)   requires ATP.

   (B)   requires a protein carrier.

   (C)   refers to the osmosis of water.

   (D)   moves substances against a concentration gradient.

   (E)   is diffusion that occurs easily.

7. A cell deprived of its series of Golgi complexes has difficulty

    (A) maintaining its shape.

    (B) synthesizing DNA.

    (C) synthesizing mRNA.

    (D) storing molecules.

    (E) synthesizing protein.

8. A cell's nucleolus is found in its

    (A) cytoplasm.

    (B) endoplasmic reticulum.

    (C) mitochondrion.

    (D) nucleus.

    (E) plasma membrane.

9. In the cytoskeleton, the _____ provide(s) the majority of the network that connects all structures in the cytoplasm.

    (A) microtrabeculae

    (B) cytoplasmic lattice

    (C) intermediate fibers

    (D) microtubules

    (E) microfilaments

10. Removal of a cell's ribosomes would result in the cell's inability to use which of the following molecules?

    (A) Carbon dioxide

    (B) Carbon monoxide

    (C) Lysine

    (D) Oxygen

    (E) Phosphorus

ANSWER KEY

1.	(C)	6.	(B)
2.	(C)	7.	(D)
3.	(C)	8.	(D)
4.	(D)	9.	(D)
5.	(A)	10.	(C)

CHAPTER 4

Tissues

4.1   Epithelium

The study of tissues is called **histology**. There are four principal kinds of tissues in the human body: epithelial tissue (epithelium), connective tissue, nervous tissue, and muscle tissue. Each major kind has a variety of subtypes.

Epithelial tissue covers the free surfaces of the body. Externally, it protects the body. As a covering for the internal surfaces, its functions range from secretion to absorption.

There are three types of epithelium based on the shape of the cells (see figure on the next page):

Squamous - Squamous cells are flat and thin.

Cuboidal - These cells are cube-shaped.

Columnar - These cells are shaped as columns, with a nucleus at the base of the cell.

Epithelium can be simple or stratified:

Simple - Simple means that the cells exist in one layer as they cover a surface.

Stratified - This means that there are many layers of epithelium covering a surface.

For example, simple squamous epithelium lines the inside of blood vessels. Simple cuboidal epithelium lines the tubules of the kidney, where the cells absorb molecules. Simple columnar epithelium lines much of the digestive tract, where it absorbs and secretes substances. Stratified squamous epithelium lines the inside of the oral cavity and composes the outer layer of the skin, the epidermis.

Other kinds of epithelium include:

Pseudostratified - It appears to be stratified, but the cells form only one layer. This tissue lines much of the respiratory tract.

Transitional - The shape of the cells changes. The epithelial cells lining the inside surface of the bladder change shape depending on the amount of urine stored.

Glandular - Glandular cells secrete. The cells of exocrine glands secrete their products into ducts. Examples are the sweat glands of the skin. Endocrine glands are ductless glands. They secrete chemical messengers, hormones, into the bloodstream.

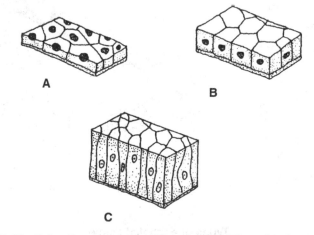

Epithelial cells: squamous (A), cuboidal (B), and columnar

Problem Solving Example:

 Describe the various types and functions of the epithelial tissues.

 Epithelial tissues form the covering or lining of the internal and external body surfaces. Epithelial tissues include, for example, the outer part of the skin, the linings of the digestive tract, the linings of the lungs, the urogenital tract, the covering of the body cavity, and so forth. The cells that make up the epithelial tissues are packed closely together, thus providing a continuous protective barrier between the underlying cells and the outside world. This protection helps to keep the body safe from mechanical injury, from harmful chemicals and bacteria, and from drying. Epithelial cells may have other functions, such as absorption, secretion, and sensation.

The surface of the epithelial cell that is exposed to air or fluid often becomes specialized. This surface commonly bears cilia, hairs, or finger-like processes. It may also be covered with waxy or mucous secretions. The opposite surface rests upon other cell layers.

ciliated columnar epithelium

cuboidal epithelium

squamous epithelium

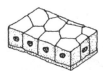

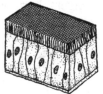

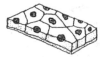

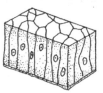

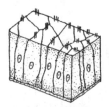

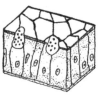

columnar epithelium

sensory epithelium

glandular epithelium

Types of epithelial tissue

Epithelial cells are generally grouped into three categories according to their shape and function: squamous, cuboidal, and columnar.

Squamous cells are much broader than they are thick and have the appearance of thin, flat plates. They are found on the surface of the skin and the lining of the mouth, esophagus, and vagina. Cuboidal epithelium (cube-shaped cells) is found in kidney tubules. The cells of columnar epithelium are long and thin, resembling pillars or columns. The stomach and intestines are lined with columnar epithelium. Some columnar cells have cilia on their surfaces. The function of the cilia is to move substances past the cell. The respiratory tract is characterized by ciliated columnar epithelium.

Epithelial tissue may further be classified as simple or stratified. Simple epithelium is one cell layer thick. Stratified epithelium consists of several layers of cells. Both simple and stratified epithelium may be squamous, cuboidal, or columnar.

4.2 Connective Tissue

Connective tissue generally consists of cells that are separated by large amounts of intercellular material that make up the matrix. There is usually an abundant supply of blood vessels throughout the matrix. The matrix may contain several types of fibers:

Collagen - These are white fibers that are flexible and tough.
Elastin - Elastin fibers are yellow and elastic.
Reticular - Reticular fibers are delicate and branching.

Connective tissue binds structures of the body. Other functions include protection, support, and insulation. There are many subtypes of connective tissue.

Areolar (Loose) Connective Tissue - This tissue contains a variety of specialized cells. **Fibroblasts** are large, star-shaped cells that produce the white and yellow fibers in the matrix. **Macrophages** are large cells that engulf debris and foreign agents in the tissue. **Mast cells** secrete heparin, an anticoagulant. **Leukocytes** (white blood cells) wander through the matrix to fight infection. **Plasma cells** produce antibodies as part of the immune system.

Areolar tissue is widespread throughout the body. It often lies beneath epithelium. It is abundant beneath the skin.

Dense Fibrous Connective Tissue - Compared to areolar connective tissue, the collagen fibers are closely packed together in dense connective tissue. The arrangement of fibers can be regular or irregular. This tissue composes the internal layer of the skin, the dermis. It is also found in tendons, which connect muscles to each other or to bones, and ligaments, which connect bones to bones.

Cartilage - The **chondrocyte** is the cartilage cell. These cells reside in depressions in the matrix, called **lacunae**. A direct blood supply is absent in cartilage. There are three subtypes based on the composition of the matrix:

Hyaline Cartilage - This tissue has fine collagen fibers. It is found in the external nose, in the wall of the trachea, and on the ends of long bones. It reduces friction between the ends of these bones.

Fibrocartilage - This tissue has tough collagen fibers. It is found in the vertebral column between the vertebrae. These wedges of cartilage serve as shock absorbers.

Elastic Cartilage - It has more elastic fibers. It is found in the external ear.

Bone - The matrix of bone tissue is fortified with salts of calcium and phosphorous, making it extremely hard. In compact bone (bone made of densely packed tissue), the **osteocytes** (bone cells) are found in lacunae. The lacunae are arranged in concentric circles around a **Haversian canal**. This canal has blood vessels and nerves serving the bone cells. Miniature canals (canaliculi) connect the lacunae with the Haversian canal for transport. This entire system is called a **Haversian system**.

Adipose - This tissue has numerous cells that store fat. It is found beneath the skin, where it serves as a layer of insulation. It is also found around the kidneys.

Blood - The **plasma** is the liquid portion of the blood. It is the matrix of this type of connective tissue. **Erythrocytes** (red blood cells) carry oxygen and carbon dioxide in the blood. **Leukocytes** (white blood cells) fight infection. **Thrombocytes** (platelets) are cell fragments that start the process of blood clotting.

Problem Solving Example:

List and compare the tissues that support and hold together the other tissues of the body.

Connective tissue supports and holds together structures of the body. It is classified into four groups by structure and/or function: bone, cartilage, blood, and fibrous connective tissue. The cells of these tissues characteristically secrete a large amount of non-cellular material, called matrix. The nature and function of each kind of connective tissue is determined largely by the nature of its matrix. Connective tissue cells are actually quite separate from each other; for most of this connective tissue, volume is made up of matrix. The cells between them function indirectly by secreting a matrix that performs the actual functions of connection or support or both.

Blood consists of erythrocytes (red blood cells), leukocytes (white blood cells), and thrombocytes (platelets) in a liquid matrix called the plasma. Blood has its major function in transporting almost any substance that is needed, anywhere in the body.

The fibrous connective tissues have a thick matrix composed of interlacing protein fibers secreted by and surrounding the connective tissue cells. These fibers are of three types: collagenous fibers, which are flexible but resist stretching and give considerable strength to the tissues containing them; elastic fibers, which can easily be stretched, but return to their normal length like a rubber band when released; and reticular fibers, which branch and interlace to form complex networks. These fibrous tissues occur throughout the body and hold skin to the muscle, keep glands in position, and bind together many other structures. Tendons and ligaments are specialized fibrous connective tissue. Tendons are not elastic but are flexible, cable-like cords that connect muscles to bones. Ligaments are semi-elastic and connect bones to bones.

The skeleton is composed of the connective tissues cartilage and bone. Cartilage cells secrete a hard, rubbery matrix around themselves. Cartilage can support great weight, yet it is flexible and somewhat elastic. Cartilage is found in the human body at the tip of the nose, in the ear flaps, larynx, trachea, intervertebral discs, on the surfaces of skeletal joints, and at the ends of ribs.

Bone has a hard, relatively rigid matrix. This matrix contains many collagenous fibers and water, both of which prevent the bone from being overly brittle. Bone is impregnated with calcium and phosphorus salts. These give bone its hardness. Bone cells that secrete the body matrix containing the calcium salts are widely separated and are located in specialized spaces in the matrix. Bone is not a solid structure, for most bones have a large marrow cavity in their centers. Also, extending through the matrix are Haversian canals, through which blood vessels and nerve fibers run in order to supply the bone cells.

4.3 Muscle Tissue

The cells of muscle tissue have the ability to shorten their length, or contract. There are three subtypes of muscle tissue: skeletal, visceral, and cardiac.

Skeletal - This tissue attaches to the bones. As it contracts, it pulls on the bones, producing body movement. The cells, called fibers, are long and thread-like. Each cell has many nuclei (multinucleated) along the inside surface of the cell membrane. Under the microscope this tissue is **striated**, meaning that it has a crossbanded appearance. It is voluntary, capable of rapid response.

Visceral - This muscle tissue is **smooth**, lacking striations, and is involuntary. The cells are small and spindle-shaped, with one nucleus per cell. This tissue is capable of slow, prolonged contractions. It composes the musculature of all internal organs except the heart. Examples include the bladder, uterus, stomach, small intestine, and middle wall of arteries and veins.

Cardiac - This tissue composes the musculature of the heart chambers. It is **striated** and involuntary. There is some branching between cells. **Intercalated disks** separate the cells transversely. Each cell has one nucleus.

Problem Solving Example:

How are the types of muscle tissues differentiated?

The cells of muscle tissue have great capacity for contraction. Muscles are able to perform work by the summed contractions of their individual cells. The individual muscle cells are usually elongated, cylindrical, or spindle-shaped cells that are bound together into sheets or bundles by connective tissue.

Three principal types of muscle tissue are found in vertebrates. Skeletal or striated muscle is responsible for most voluntary movements. Visceral or smooth muscle is involved in most involuntary movements of internal organs, such as the stomach. Cardiac muscle is the tissue of which much of the heart wall is composed; it is also involuntary.

Most skeletal muscle, as the name implies, is attached to the bones of the body, and its contraction is responsible for the movements of parts of the skeleton. Skeletal muscle contraction is also involved in other activities of the body, such as the voluntary release of urine and feces. Thus, the movements produced by skeletal muscle are primarily involved with interactions between the body and the external environment.

Skeletal muscle reveals a striated appearance, and is therefore also referred to as striated muscle. These striations are actually due to the regular arrangement of thick and thin myofilaments in individual muscle fiber cells. Skeletal muscle is an exception to the common observation that each cell contains only one nucleus; each skeletal fiber cell is multinucleated. Skeletal muscle can contract very rapidly but cannot remain contracted; the fibers must relax before the next contraction can occur.

Comparison of the Types of Muscle Tissue

	Skeletal	Smooth	Cardiac
Location	Attached to skeleton	Walls of visceral organs, walls of blood vessels	Walls of heart
Shape of fiber	Elongated, cylindrical, blunt ends	Elongated, spindle-shaped, pointed ends	Elongated, cylindrical, fibers branch and fuse
Number of nuclei per fiber	Many	One	Many
Position of nuclei	Peripheral	Central	Central
Cross striations	Present	Absent	Present
Speed of contractions	Most rapid	Slowest	Intermediate
Ability to remain contracted	Least	Greatest	Intermediate
Type of control	Voluntary	Involuntary	Involuntary

Visceral muscle can be classified as smooth muscle. It is found in the walls of hollow visceral organs, such as the uterus, urinary bladder, bronchioles, and much of the gastrointestinal tract. Vascular smooth muscle refers to that smooth muscle in the walls of blood vessels. Unlike skeletal muscle cells that are cylindrical, multinucleate, and striated, smooth muscle cells are spindle-shaped, uninucleate, and lack striations. This lack of striations accounts for its smooth appearance. Smooth muscle cells have a slower speed of contraction, but can remain contracted for a longer period of time than the striated muscle cells.

Cardiac muscle has properties similar to those of both skeletal and smooth muscles. Like skeletal muscle cells, cardiac muscle cells are striated. Like smooth muscle fibers, cardiac muscle fibers are uninucleated and are designed for endured contractions rather than speedy or strong contractions. Cardiac and smooth muscles are not voluntarily controlled but have spontaneous activities and are regulated by the autonomic nervous system. The skeletal muscle, being voluntary, is controlled by the somatic nervous system.

4.4 Nerve Tissue

The **neuron** is the specialized cell of nerve tissue. It has the ability to send signals. The signal normally travels from the **dendrites** to the **cell body** to the **axon** of the nerve cell. The cell body contains the nucleus and most of the cytoplasm. The dendrites and axon are processes, or nerve fibers, of the cell. Outside the brain and spinal cord (central nervous system), these processes are found in nerves. Nerves send messages from sense organs to the central nervous system and also send them in the opposite direction to organs that make responses (e.g., skeletal muscles).

Glial cells are another type of cell in nerve tissue. They protect and support nerves.

Problem Solving Example:

Which tissue in the body is responsible for the rapid transmission of information?

To some extent, all cells have the property of irritability, the ability to respond to stimuli. Nervous tissue, however, is highly specialized not only for receiving and responding to such stimuli, but also for the transmission of stimuli. Nerve cells are easily stimulated and can transmit impulses very rapidly. Each nerve cell is specific for the type of information it transmits, and the impulse is directed and coordinated to specific areas in the body.

Nervous tissue consists of neurons, cells that conduct electrochemical nerve impulses. Each neuron has an enlarged cell body, which contains the nucleus and two or more thin, hair-like processes extending from the

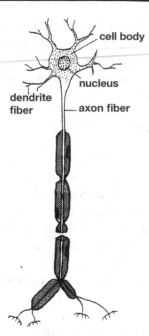

Nerve cell. The dendrites carry impulses toward the cell body. The axon carries impulses away from the cell body.

cell body. There are two distinct types of these processes; they differ in the direction they normally conduct a nerve impulse. Axons conduct nerve impulses away from the cell body, while dendrites conduct impulses toward the cell body. The neurons are connected together in chains or networks in order to relay impulses for long distances to different parts of the body. The junction between the terminals of the axon of one neuron and the dendrite of the next neuron in line is called a synapse. The axon and dendrite do not actually touch at the synapse. There is a small gap between the two processes. An impulse can travel across the synapse only in one direction, from an axon to a dendrite. In this way the synapse functions in preventing impulses from backflowing in the wrong direction. A group of axons bound together by connective tissue constitutes a nerve. The functional combination of nerve and muscle tissue is fundamental to the human body. These tissues give the characteristic ability to move rapidly in response to stimuli. In other words, muscle contraction, and thus movement, are initiated and controlled by nervous tissue.

CHAPTER 5

The Skin

5.1 Functions

The skin is a widespread organ, representing about 3,000 square inches of body surface. It consists of the **epidermis** (outer layer) and **dermis** (inner layer). Its functions include protection, sensory reception, regulation of body temperature, vitamin D synthesis, and identification.

Protection - The skin provides a barrier that protects the entire body. It offers a line of defense against invading bacteria. It serves as a cushion to guard underlying structures from physical forces striking the body. The skin is waterproofed by a thin, oily film secreted by sebaceous glands. Melanin is a dark pigment found in the cells of the epidermis. This pigment screens out ultraviolet rays from the sun that can damage tissues.

Sensory Reception - Receptors are specialized cells that detect environmental changes called stimuli. The layers of the skin contain receptors for touch, pressure, pain, and temperature. Sensory neurons in the skin send signals from receptors to the central nervous system for interpretation.

Regulation of Body Temperature - The dermis contains an abundant supply of blood vessels. The blood carries body heat. If the cutaneous (skin) vessels supplying the skin dilate, more blood reaches the surface of the body through the skin. The heat can escape from these dilated blood vessels. This response serves as a cooling mechanism. If these supplying vessels constrict, less blood reaches the surface of the body for heat liberation. This response conserves body heat.

The skin also contains sweat glands. As these glands secrete perspiration, heat is required to evaporate this substance from the body surface. This heat is supplied from the body. Therefore, this response cools the body as heat is liberated.

Vitamin D Synthesis - Ultraviolet rays stimulate the synthesis of vitamin D by skin cells. Vitamin D is converted to other substances that regulate the storage of calcium and phosphorous in the bones.

Identification - Papillae are ridges where the epidermis and dermis meet. On the surface these ridges appear as fingerprints and palm prints, which are individually distinctive and can be used for identification purposes.

Problem Solving Example:

Q The skin is much more than merely an outer wrapping; it is an important organ system and performs many diverse functions. What are some of the primary functions of the skin in humans?

A Perhaps the most vital function of the skin is to protect the body against a variety of external agents and to maintain a constant internal environment. The layers of the skin form a protective shield against blows, friction, and many injurious chemicals. These layers are essentially germproof, and as long as they are not broken, keep bacteria and other microorganisms from entering the body. The skin is water-repellent and therefore protects the body from excessive loss of moisture. In addition, the pigment in the outer layers protects the underlying layers from the ultraviolet rays of the sun.

In addition to its role in protection, the skin is involved in thermoregulation. Heat is constantly being produced by the metabolic processes of the body cells and distributed by the bloodstream. Heat may be lost from the body in expired breath, feces, and urine, but approximately 90 percent of the total heat loss occurs through the skin. This is accomplished by changes in the blood supply to the capillaries in the skin. When the air temperature and body temperature are high, the skin capillaries dilate, and the increased flow of blood results in increased heat loss. Due to the increased blood supply, the skin appears flushed. When the temperature is low, the arterioles of the skin are constricted, thereby decreasing the flow of blood through the skin and decreasing the rate of heat loss. Temperature-sensitive nerve endings in the skin reflexively control arteriole diameters.

At high temperatures, the sweat glands are stimulated to secrete sweat. The evaporation of sweat from the surface of the skin lowers the body temperature by removing from the body the heat necessary to convert the liquid sweat into water vapor. In addition to their function in heat loss, the sweat glands also serve an excretory function. Five to ten percent of all metabolic wastes are excreted by the sweat glands. Sweat contains similar substances as urine but is much more dilute.

5.2 Structure

The skin is an organ consisting of several tissues (see figure on the next page). Stratified squamous epithelium composes the outer layer of the skin, the epidermis. Dense connective tissue composes the deeper, thicker layer of the skin, the dermis. A subcutaneous layer is found beneath the dermis. It is composed of areolar connective tissue and adipose tissue. Sometimes it is counted as a third layer of the skin and called the hypodermis.

5.2.1 Epidermis

The epidermis consists of four or five sublayers depending on its location in the body. The layers range from the outermost sublayer, the stratum corneum, to the deepest layer, the stratum basale. Each layer forms cells that become part of the sublayer next to it externally.

The **stratum corneum** consists of squamous epithelial cells that are dead. The cells of this sublayer are cornified, meaning that they are hard and filled with the protein keratin. The cells are dead because they are too far from the nutrients and oxygen supplied from the blood found in the underlying dermis. Therefore, they are constantly being shed from the body surface. Division by cells in the deeper sublayers of the epidermis replace the cells in this layer as they are lost.

The **stratum lucidium** is present if five sublayers are present where the skin is thicker. Examples include the palms of hands, fingertips, and soles of feet. When present, this sublayer of dead cells is under the stratum corneum.

The **stratum granulosum** consists of flattened epithelial cells. As these cells are pushed toward the surface, they gradually lose their organelles and die.

The **stratum spinosum** consists of living cells under the stratum granulosum. As they divide, they are pushed toward the granulosum.

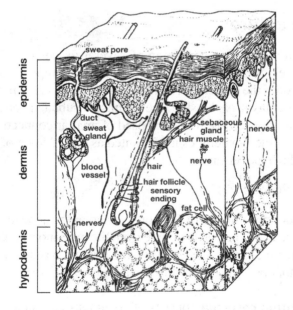

Section of the skin: epidermis, dermis, and hypodermis

The **stratum basale** is the deepest sublayer of the epidermis. It is a single layer of column-shaped cells that are actively dividing. New cells produced are pushed outward, where they become part of the stratum spinosum.

5.2.2 Dermis

The dermis contains numerous structures. Many of the functions of the skin are determined by the action of these structures.

The dermis is laced with **collagen** and **elastin** fibers. The collagen provides toughness and the elastin fibers allow the skin to stretch.

Arteries supply blood to the dermis. **Veins** transport blood away from this layer. If the capillaries dilate, more blood is supplied to the dermis. This blood carries heat that can escape from the body. If the supplying vessels constrict, body heat is conserved; therefore, this blood flow contributes to temperature regulation.

The dermis contains numerous **neurons** and **receptors**. Through these structures, the skin serves as a sensory organ. There are different receptors specialized for different stimuli: touch, pressure, pain, and temperature. Sensory neurons conduct signals from these receptors to the central nervous system.

Sweat glands form and secrete perspiration. The ducts of these exocrine glands extend from the epidermis to the skin surface. The secretion and evaporation of perspiration serve as a cooling mechanism.

Where hair is present in the skin, the root of each hair is anchored in a chamber called the **hair follicle**. **Sebaceous glands** are associated with these hair follicles. These glands secrete an oily product, sebum, that covers and waterproofs the skin surface.

Small masses of smooth muscle tissue, the **arrector pili** muscles, are also associated with the hair follicles. They contract when external temperatures are cold, producing the familiar "goosebumps."

Papillae are the ridges at the boundary of the dermis and stratum basale of the epidermis. These ridges are pronounced enough to establish fingerprints and palmprints.

Problem Solving Example:

Q The skin consists of many layers of cells. It is the largest organ of the human body. Describe the major physical characteristics of skin. What structures are derived from human skin?

A Human skin is composed of a comparatively thin, outer layer, the epidermis, which is free of blood vessels, and an inner, thick layer, the dermis, which is packed with blood vessels and nerve endings. The epidermis is a stratified epithelium whose thickness varies in different parts of the body. It is thickest on the soles of the feet and the palms of the hands. The epidermis of the palms and fingers has numerous ridges, forming whorls and loops in very specific patterns. These unique fingerprints and palm prints are determined genetically, and result primarily from the orientation of the underlying fibers in the dermis. The outermost layers of the epidermis are composed of dead cells that are constantly being sloughed off and replaced by cells from beneath. As each cell is pushed outward by active cell division in the deeper layers of the epidermis, it is compressed into a flat (squamous), scale-like epithelial cell. Such cells synthesize large amounts of the fibrous protein keratin, which serves to toughen the epidermis and make it more durable.

Scattered at the juncture between the deeper layers of the epidermis and the dermis are melanocytes, cells that produce the pigment melanin. Melanin serves as a protective device for the body by absorbing ultraviolet rays from the sun. Tanning results from an increase in melanin production as a result of exposure to ultraviolet radiation. All humans have about the same number of melanocytes in their skin. The difference between light- and dark-skinned races is under genetic control and occurs because melanocytes of dark-skinned races produce more melanin.

The juncture of the dermis with the epidermis is uneven. The dermis throws projections called papillae into the epidermis. The dermis is much thicker than the epidermis and is composed largely of connective tissue. The subcutaneous layer, below the dermis, is connected with the underlying muscle and is composed of many fat cells and a more loosely woven network of fibers. This part of the dermis is one of the principal sites of body fat deposits, which help preserve body heat. The subcutaneous layer also determines the amount of possible skin movement.

The hair and nails are derivatives of skin and develop from inpocketings of cells from the inner layer of the epidermis. Hair follicles are found throughout the entire dermal layer, except on the palms, soles, and a few other regions. Individual hairs are formed in the hair follicles, which have their roots deep within the dermis. At the bottom of each follicle, a papilla of connective tissue projects into the follicle. The epithelial cells above this papilla constitute the hair root and, by cell division, form the shaft of the hair, which ultimately extends beyond the surface of the skin. The hair cells of the shaft secrete keratin, then die and form a compact mass that becomes hair. Growth occurs at the bottom of the follicle only. Associated with each hair follicle is one or more sebaceous glands, the secretions of which make the surface of the skin and hair more pliable. Like the sweat glands, the sebaceous glands are derived from the embryonic epidermis but are located in the dermis. To each hair follicle is attached smooth muscle called arrector pili, which pulls the hair erect upon contraction.

Nails grow in a manner similar to hair. Both hair follicles and nails develop from inpocketings of cells from the inner layer of the epidermis. The translucent, densely packed, dead cells of the nails allow the underlying capillaries to show through and give the nails their normal pink color.

5.3   Accessory Structures

Accessory structures originate from the layers of the skin. These include the glands (sweat and sebaceous), hair, and nails. The toenails and fingernails consist of a specialized, hardened type of keratin that is produced from epidermal cells.

The skin is often called the integument. The integument and accessory structures are recognized as one of the organ systems of the body, the **integumentary system**.

5.4 Membranes

Membranes are large, sheet-like boundaries that cover the surfaces of the body. There are four kinds of membranes: cutaneous, mucous, serous, and synovial. Each membrane consists of an epithelial tissue mounted on a base of connective tissue.

Cutaneous Membrane - The skin is the cutaneous membrane. Stratified squamous epithelium composes the epidermis. Dense connective tissue composes the dermis.

Mucous Membrane - Mucous membranes line the internal body cavities that are contiguous with the external environment. Examples include the respiratory, digestive, urinary, and reproductive tracts. The epithelial cells of these membranes secrete mucous, which prevents the drying out of the membrane. It also offers lubrication.

Serous Membrane - Serous membranes line body cavities and organs that are sealed off from the external environment.

Serous membranes usually exist at two levels. The **parietal** membrane lines the cavity. The **visceral** membrane lines the organ within the cavity. For example, the parietal pleura is a serous membrane that lines the part of the thoracic cavity around the lung. The visceral pleura (pulmonary pleura) adheres to the lung surface. These membranes seal off a cavity around each lung, the pleural (intrapleural) cavity.

Synovial Membrane - Synovial membranes line the cavities of joint capsules at the freely movable joints. These secrete an oily product, synovium, which serves as a lubricant.

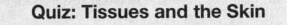

Quiz: Tissues and the Skin

1. Simple squamous tissue is a type of which of the following kinds of tissue?

    (A) Connective   (D) Nerve

    (B) Epithelial   (E) Vascular

    (C) Muscle

2. Which of the following tissues is NOT related to connective tissue?

    (A) Blood   (D) Lymph

    (B) Bone   (E) Collagen

    (C) Cartilage

3. The skin performs all of the following human body functions EXCEPT

    (A) identification of an individual.

    (B) protection.

    (C) sensation.

    (D) storage.

    (E) temperature regulation.

4. The extracellular fibers found in all connective tissues are composed mainly of

    (A) collagen.   (D) glycans.

    (B) calcium.   (E) Both (A) and (C).

    (C) elastin.

5. The tissue that lines the inside of blood vessels is known as

   (A) epithelial tissue.

   (B) connective tissue.

   (C) adipose tissue.

   (D) hyaline cartilage.

   (E) reticular tissue.

6. Which tissue has the ability to repair itself most rapidly?

   (A) Epithelium   (D) Nerve

   (B) Connective   (E) Bone

   (C) Muscle

7. All of the following are true of skeletal muscle EXCEPT

   (A) muscle fibers are long and thread-like.

   (B) each cell is multinucleated.

   (C) it comprises the middle walls of arteries and veins.

   (D) it is attached to bone.

   (E) the tissue is striated.

8. Smooth muscle is found in which of the following subtypes of muscle tissue?

   (A) Skeletal

   (B) Visceral

   (C) Cardiac

   (D) All of the above.

   (E) None of the above.

9. A signal travels through a nerve in the following order:

   (A) dendrite, cell body, axon.

   (B) dendrite, axon, cell body.

   (C) cell body, axon, dendrite.

   (D) axon, cell body, dendrite.

   (E) axon, dendrite, cell body.

10. Glial cells are part of which of the following kinds of tissue?

   (A) Muscle

   (B) Nerve

   (C) Connective

   (D) Adipose

   (E) Epithelial

ANSWER KEY

1.	(B)	6.	(A)
2.	(D)	7.	(C)
3.	(D)	8.	(B)
4.	(E)	9.	(A)
5.	(A)	10.	(B)

CHAPTER 6

The Skeletal System

6.1 Functions

The skeletal system consists of 206 bones that are large enough to be counted. It provides at least five functions for the human body.

Protection - Many organs are contained within spaces formed by the bones. The cranium, which is the superior portion of the skull, houses the brain. The vertebral column surrounds the spinal cord. Twelve pairs of ribs and the sternum, composing the thoracic cage, protect many organs in the central body cavity. Examples include the heart, lungs, stomach, and liver.

Support - The vertebral column has four different curvatures along its length. These curvatures give the backbone a great ability to support body weight. The arch formed by the bones of the foot also supports body weight. Other bones, such as the long bones in the legs and arms, contribute great mechanical strength.

Movement - Skeletal muscles attach to the bones. As the muscles contract, they pull on the bones and produce movement. For example, the forearm bones (radius and ulna) are pulled toward the upper arm bone (humerus) as the biceps brachii muscle contracts. The forearm bones and humerus are connected by a hinge joint. This joint permits the bending (flexion) of the forearm when the biceps muscle in the upper arm contracts.

Mineral Storage - Calcium and phosphorous are stored in the bones. If the concentration of these minerals is too high in the blood, the excess amount is stored in the bones. If more of these minerals is needed in the blood, they are released from the bones.

Blood Cell Formation (Hemopoiesis) - The bones are not solid structures. Cavities in the cranial bones, vertebrae, ribs, sternum, and ends of long bones contain red marrow. This blood-forming tissue produces erythrocytes (red blood cells), leukocytes (white blood cells), and thrombocytes (platelets). From these sites of production, these cells are released into the circulation.

Problem Solving Example:

 Besides their function in locomotion and support, bones also serve several other important functions. What are they?

Bones are an important reservoir for certain minerals. The mineral content of bones is constantly being renewed. Roughly all the mineral content of bone is removed and replaced every nine months. Calcium and phosphorus are especially abundant in the bones and must be maintained in the blood at a constant level. When the diet is low in these minerals, they can be withdrawn from the bones to maintain the proper concentration in the blood. Stress on the bone seems to be necessary for the maintenance of calcium and phosphate in the bones, for in the absence of stress these minerals pass from the bones into the blood faster than they are taken in. This elevates the blood concentration of these minerals to a very high level, which may ultimately lead to the development of kidney stones. Before special stress exercise programs were developed, astronauts in space often became victims of this type of kidney trouble.

During pregnancy, when the demand for minerals to form bones of a growing fetus is great, a woman's own bones may become depleted unless her diet contains more of these minerals than is normally needed. During starvation, the blood can draw on the storehouse of minerals in the bones and maintain life much longer than would be possible without this means of storage. Bones are also important in that they give rise to the fundamental elements of the circulatory system.

Bone marrow is the site of production of lymphocyte precursor cells, which play an integral role in the body's immune response system. Red blood cells, or erythrocytes, also originate in the bone marrow. As erythrocytes mature, they accumulate hemoglobin, the oxygen carrier of blood. Mature erythrocytes, however, are incomplete cells lacking nuclei and the metabolic machinery to synthesize new protein. They are released into the bloodstream where they circulate for approximately 120 days before being destroyed by phagocytes. Thus, the bone marrow must perform the constant task of maintaining the level of erythrocytes for the packaging of hemoglobin.

6.2   Growth and Development

Based on shape, there are five kinds of bones that develop in the body. **Long** bones are found in the arms (e.g., humerus, the upper arm bone) and legs (e.g., femur, the thighbone). **Short** bones include the carpals (wrist) and tarsals (ankle). Some bones are **flat**, such as the sternum. Others are **irregular**, such as the mandible (jawbone) and vertebrae. **Sesamoid** bones are seed-shaped, found in joints (e.g., patella, the kneecap bone).

Long bones increase in diameter through the activity of cells. Cells called **osteoblasts** on the surface of the bone produce layers of new bone cells, **osteocytes**. These bone cells mature and produce a matrix, surrounding inorganic material, to increase the amount of compact (dense) bone tissue. As this process progresses, the long bone increases in diameter.

The activity of osteoblasts and osteocytes also produces compact bone tissue in the other kinds of bones (short, flat, irregular, and sesamoid).

Long bones also increase in length during growth and development. The **epiphyseal plate** (disc) is a wedge of cartilage accounting for this increase. This plate is found between the epiphysis (bulbous end) and diaphysis (tubular shaft) at each end of the bone. The cartilage cells of the epiphyseal plate form layers of compact bone tissue, adding to the length of the bone. This disc becomes inactive in most individuals by the late teens or early twenties.

In the adult, the skeletal system is constantly being remodeled. Bones are being broken down and rebuilt. **Osteoclasts** are cells that break down and remove exhausted bone tissue. Osteoblasts build new bone tissue to replace this loss.

Problem Solving Example:

Q Bone, like other connective tissues, consists of cells and fibers; its extracellular components are calcified, making it a hard, unyielding substance ideally suited for its supportive and protective function in the skeleton. Describe the macroscopic and microscopic structure of bone.

A Upon inspection of a long bone with the naked eye, two forms of bone are distinguishable: cancellous (spongy) and compact. Spongy bone consists of a network of hardened bars having spaces between them filled with marrow. Compact bone appears as a solid, continuous mass, in which spaces can be seen only with the aid of a microscope. The two forms of bone grade into one another without a sharp boundary (see figure on the next page).

In typical long bones, such as the femur or humerus, the shaft (diaphysis) consists of compact bone surrounding a large central marrow cavity composed of spongy bone. In adults, the marrow in the long bones is primarily of the yellow, fatty variety, while the marrow in the flat bones of the ribs and at the ends of long bones is primarily of the red variety and is active in the production of red blood cells. Even this red marrow contains about 70 percent fat.

The ends (epiphysis) of long bones consist mainly of spongy bone covered by a thin layer of compact bone. This region of the long bones contains a cartilaginous region known as an epiphyseal plate. The epiphyseal cartilage and the adjacent spongy bone constitute a growth zone, in which all growth in length of the bone occurs. The surfaces at

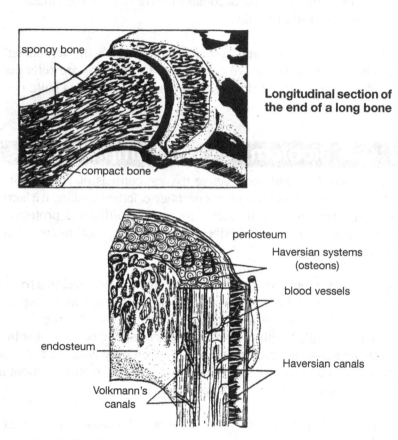

Longitudinal section of the end of a long bone

Cross section of a long bone showing internal structures

the ends of long bones, where one bone articulates with another, are covered by a layer of cartilage, called the articular cartilage. It is this cartilage that allows for easy movement of the bones over each other at a joint.

Compact bone is composed of structural units called Haversian systems. Each system is irregularly cylindrical and is composed of concentrically arranged layers of hard, inorganic matrix surrounding a microscopic central Haversian canal. Blood vessels and nerves pass through this canal, supplying and controlling the metabolism of the bone cells. The bone matrix itself is laid down by bone cells called osteoblasts. Osteoblasts produce a substance, osteoid, which is hardened by calcium, causing calcification. Some osteoblasts are trapped in the hardening osteoid and are converted into osteocytes, which continue to live within the bone. These osteocytes lie in small cavities called lacunae, located along the interfaces between adjoining concentric layers of the hard matrix. Exchange of materials between the bone cells and the blood vessels in the Haversian canals is by way of radiating canals. Other canals, known as Volkmann's canals, penetrate and cross the layers of hard matrix, connecting the different Haversian canals to one another (see figure on the previous page).

With few exceptions, bones are covered by the periosteum, a layer of specialized connective tissue. The periosteum has the ability to form bone and contributes to the healing of fractures. Periosteum is lacking on ends of long bones which are surrounded by articular cartilage. The marrow cavity of the diaphysis and the cavities of spongy bone are lined by the endosteum, a thin cellular layer that also has the ability to form bone (osteogenic potencies).

Haversian-type systems are present in most compact bone; however, certain compact flat bones of the skull (the frontal, parietal, occipital, and temporal bones, and part of the mandible) do not have Haversian systems. These bones, termed membrane bones, have a different architecture and are formed differently than bones with Haversian systems.

6.3   Gross Anatomy of a Long Bone

A long bone, such as the femur, can be used to illustrate the gross (large) anatomy of a bone. Its major parts include:

Epiphysis - Bulb-like end proximally and distally.

Diaphysis - Tube-like shaft between the epiphyses.

Metaphysis - Line between the epiphysis and diaphysis—this is the earlier site of the epiphyseal plate during bone growth.

Medullary Cavity - A cavity in the diaphysis; this is filled with yellow marrow in the adult. Yellow marrow is mainly fat tissue.

Compact Bone - Dense bone tissue composing the wall of the diaphysis.

Cancellous Bone - Spongy bone tissue in the epiphysis—the spaces of this spongy bone are filled with red marrow that produces blood cells.

Endosteum - The lining of the medullary cavity.

Periosteum - The outer covering on the diaphysis—it is necessary for the nutritional maintenance of the long bone.

Articular Cartilage - Hyaline cartilage covering the ends of the long bone at the joints (articulations)—this smooth covering reduces friction during movement.

6.4   Microscopic Anatomy of a Bone

Compact bone tissue is a type of connective tissue. The matrix of this tissue consists mainly of collagen plus salts of calcium and phosphorous. These mineralized salts give the matrix the characteristics of reinforced concrete.

In addition to the matrix, compact bone consists of:

Osteocytes - The bone cells.

Lacunae - Each lacuna is a depression in the matrix where an osteocyte is located.

Lamellae - Each lamella is a circular layer of osteocytes located in lacunae.

Canaliculi - Processes connecting the lacunae—each canaliculus resembles a miniature canal.

Haversian Canal - This is a central canal around which the concentric lamellae are located. The Haversian canal contains blood vessels and nerves that serve the osteocytes. Exchange of substances (e.g., oxygen, nutrients) between the central canal and osteocytes occurs along the canaliculi connecting the lacunae to the Haversian canal.

The Haversian canal and surrounding structures form a **Haversian system**. This repeating system is found in the compact bone of the diaphysis of a long bone.

Cancellous bone tissue is found in the epiphyses of long bones and inside the short, flat, irregular, and sesamoid bones. It consists of interconnecting plates called **trabeculae**. Each trabecula consists of several lamellae with osteocytes.

Problem Solving Example:

Q Bone always develops by replacement of a preexisting connective tissue. When bone formation takes place in preexisting cartilage it is called endochondral ossification. Describe this method of bone formation.

A Bones at the base of the skull, in the vertebral column, the pelvis, and the limbs are called cartilage bones because they originate from cartilage. This cartilage, present in the infant, is replaced with bone in later years by means of a process called endochondral ossification. This can best be studied in one of the long bones of an extremity. We first start with a cartilaginous shaft. This shaft begins to ossify, or harden into bone, around its midportion, due to the deposition of calcium by the cartilage cells (chondrocytes). At the same time, blood vessels from the surrounding layer of connective tissue grow into the diaphysis. The calcified cartilage cells then die and are replaced by cells called osteoblasts, which form the bone matrix. The thin-walled blood vessels branch and grow toward either end of the cartilage model, forming capillary loops that extend into the blind ends of the cavities in the calcified cartilage. Cells are brought into the interior of the cartilage by these vessels. These cells later form bone marrow or bone matrix.

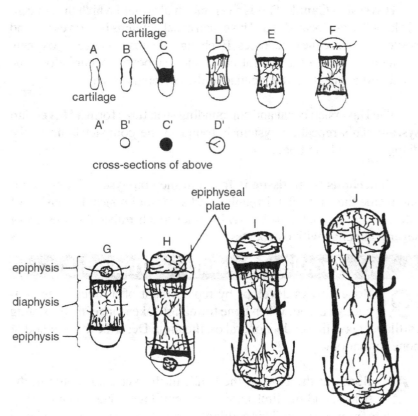

Schematic diagram showing the growth of a long bone

In the continuing growth in length, the cartilage cells in the epiphyses become arranged in longitudinal columns. The epiphyses, like the diaphyses before them, are invaded by blood vessels and begin undergoing ossification. The expansion of these centers of ossification gradually replaces all of the epiphyseal cartilage except that which persists as the articular cartilage and a transverse disk of longitudinal columns of cartilage between the original area of ossification and the epiphyseal area of ossification, called the epiphyseal plate. The epiphyseal plate contains the cartilage columns in which the zone of proliferation is responsible for all subsequent growth in length in long bones. Under normal conditions, the rate of multiplication of cartilage cells in this zone is in balance with their rate of replacement by bone. The epiphyseal plate, therefore, retains approximately the same thickness. Growth in length is the result of the cartilage cells continually growing away from the shaft and being replaced by bone as they recede. The net result is an increase in the length of the shaft. At the end of the growing period, proliferation of cartilage cells slows and finally ceases. The remaining cartilage becomes converted to bone, and it is at this point that no further growth in length can occur.

The growth in diameter of bone does not depend upon the calcification of cartilage but rather is the result of deposition of new bone by the periosteum.

6.5 Axial Skeleton

The axial skeleton is one branch of the skeletal system. It forms the midline of the skeleton. This branch consists of the skull, hyoid bone, vertebral column, and thoracic cage. Eighty of the 206 bones of the skeleton are axial.

Skull - Twenty-eight bones are found in the skull. Eight bones make up the **cranium** or superior portion of the skull. They are the **frontal, temporal (2), parietal (2), occipital, ethmoid**, and **sphenoid** bones. The cranium houses the brain.

The 14 bones of the face are the **maxillae (2), zygomatic (2), nasal (2), lacrimal (2), palatine (2), inferior nasal conchae (2), vomer**, and **mandible** (jawbone). The mandible is the only movable bone of the skull. All others are connected by immovable joints called sutures. Three middle-ear bones are found in each temporal bone.

Hyoid Bone - This is a horseshoe-shaped bone suspended by muscles and ligaments from the floor of the oral cavity.

Vertebral Column - The backbone consists of four curvatures: **cervical** (neck), **thoracic** (chest), **lumbar** (lower back), and **pelvic**. Each consists of a serial arrangement of vertebrae. These vertebrae form a continuous tube, housing the spinal cord.

The cervical curvature has seven vertebrae. The **atlas** is the first cervical vertebra (C1), supporting the skull. The **axis** is the second cervical vertebra (C2). The seventh cervical vertebra is the most inferior.

Twelve thoracic vertebrae compose the thoracic curvature. The first thoracic vertebra is most superior. The 12th vertebra is the most inferior one.

Five lumbar vertebrae make up the lumbar curvature. From the base of the brain, the spinal cord inside the backbone ends inferiorly at the first lumbar vertebra. The **sacrum** (five fused vertebrae) and **coccyx** (tailbone—four, or possibly five, fused vertebrae) make up the pelvic curvature. The sacrum is directly under the fifth lumbar vertebra. The coccyx is the most inferior part of the vertebral column.

Discs of fibrocartilage (**intervertebral discs**) are found between the bodies (anterior portions) of the vertebrae. They act as shock absorbers, adding springiness to the backbone. **Intervertebral foramina** between the vertebrae are openings for the passage of blood vessels and spinal nerves communicating with the spinal cord.

Thoracic Cage - The thoracic cage consists of the **sternum** and 12 pairs of **ribs**. The sternum (breastbone) consists of three pieces: **manubrium** (most superior), **body**, and **xiphoid process** (most inferior).

Each rib pair (1 through 12) articulates posteriorly with the thoracic vertebra (12) of the same number. Anteriorly, the **vertebrosternal** ribs (1 through 7) articulate with the sternum. The **vertebrochondral** ribs (8 through 10) articulate with the cartilage connecting rib pair 7 with the sternum. The **vertebral** ribs (11 and 12) articulate only with the vertebrae.

Rib pairs 1 through 7 are also called the **true** ribs. Rib pairs 8 through 12 are called the **false** ribs.

6.6   Appendicular Skeleton

The appendicular skeleton is the other branch of the skeletal system. It contains 126 bones. This branch consists of the **pectoral** (chest) **girdle** and arm bones as well as the **pelvic** (hip) **girdle** and leg bones.

Pectoral Girdle - Each half of the pectoral girdle consists of the **clavicle** (collarbone) and **scapula** (shoulder blade). The medial end of the clavicle articulates to the manubrium of the sternum. Laterally, it attaches to the acromion of the scapula.

Arm Bones - The **humerus** is the upper arm bone. The head at the proximal end of each humerus articulates with the glenoid fossa, a shallow depression of the scapula.

In anatomical position, the **radius** is the lateral bone of each forearm. The **ulna** is the medial forearm bone.

Each wrist consists of eight **carpal** bones, a proximal and distal row of four each.

The **metacarpals** are five bones in the palm of each hand.

The **phalanges** (singular, phalanx) are the bones of the fingers. Two are in the thumb. Three are in each of the other fingers.

Pelvic Girdle - The pelvic girdle consists of the two **os coxa** or hip bones. They connect anteriorly by a slightly movable joint, the **symphysis pubis**. Combined posteriorly with the sacrum and coccyx of the axial skeleton, they form the **pelvis**.

Leg Bones - The **femur** is the thigh bone. The head at the proximal end of each femur fits into the acetabulum, a shallow depression of the hip bone. Distally, the femur joins the tibia (shinbone).

The **patella** is the kneecap bone. Each is connected distally to the tibia by a ligament. Proximally, it attaches to the quadriceps muscle on the front of the thigh by a tendon.

The **tibia** is the thicker, medial bone of each calf. The **fibula** is the lateral, thinner bone.

Seven **tarsal** bones compose each ankle and the posterior portion of the foot.

Five **metatarsals** compose the arch of each foot.

The **phalanges** are the bones of the toes. Two are in the big toe. Three are found in each of the other toes.

Problem Solving Example:

Q The vertebrate skeleton may be divided into two general parts: the axial skeleton and the appendicular skeleton. Which bones constitute these in humans?

A The axial skeleton consists of the skull, vertebral column, ribs, sternum, and hyoid bone. The primary function of the vertebrate skull is the protection of the brain. The part of the skull that serves this function is the cranium. The rest of the skull is made up of the bones of the face. In all, the human skull is composed of 28 bones, six of which are very small and located in the middle ear. At the time of birth, several of the bones of the cranium are not completely formed, leaving five membranous regions called fontanels. These regions are somewhat flexible and can undergo changes in shape as necessary for safe passage of the infant through the birth canal.

The human vertebral column, or spine, is made up of 33 separate bones known as vertebrae, which differ in size and shape in different

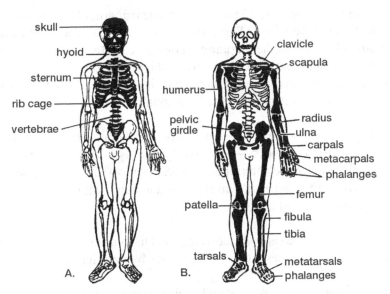

Diagram of human showing (A) the bones of the axial skeleton and (B) the bones of the appendicular skeleton

regions of the spine. In the neck region there are seven cervical vertebrae; in the thorax there are twelve thoracic vertebrae; in the lower back region there are five lumbar vertebrae; in the sacral or hip region, five fused vertebrae form the sacrum to which the pelvic girdle is attached; and at the end of the vertebral column is the coccyx or tailbone, which consists of four, or possibly five, small fused vertebrae. The vertebrae forming the sacrum and coccyx are separate in childhood, with fusion occurring by adulthood. The coccyx is a vestige of a tail in humans.

A typical vertebra consists of a basal portion, the centrum, and a dorsal ring of bone, the neural arch, which surrounds and protects the delicate spinal cord that runs through it. Each vertebra has projections for the attachment of ribs or muscles or both and for articulating (joining) with neighboring vertebrae. The first vertebra, the atlas, has rounded depressions on its upper surface into which fit two projections from the base of the skull. This articulation allows for up and down movements of the head. The second vertebra, called the axis, has a pointed projection that fits into the atlas. This type of articulation allows for the rotation of the head.

In humans, there are 12 pairs of ribs, one pair articulating with each of the thoracic vertebrae. These ribs support the chest wall and keep it from collapsing as the diaphragm contracts. Of the 12 pairs of ribs, the first seven are attached ventrally to the breastbone; the next three are attached indirectly by cartilage; and the last two, called "floating ribs," have no attachments to the breastbone.

The sternum or breastbone consists of three bones—the manubrium, body, and xiphoid process—that usually fuse by middle age. The sternum is the site for the anterior attachment of most of the ribs. The ribs and sternum together make up the thoracic cage, which functions to protect the heart and lungs.

The hyoid bone supports the tongue and its muscles. It has no articulation with other bones, but is held in place by muscles and ligaments.

The bones of the girdles and their appendages make up the appendicular skeleton. In the shoulder region the pectoral girdle, which is generally larger in males than in females, serves for the attachment of the forelimbs. The pectoral girdle consists of two collarbones, or clavicles, and two shoulder blades, or scapulas. In the hip region, the pelvic girdle serves for the attachment of the hindlimbs. The pelvic girdle, which is wider in females to allow room for fetal development, consists of three fused hipbones, called the ilium, ischium, and pubis, which are attached to the sacrum.

Articulating with the scapula is the single bone of the upper arm, called the humerus. Articulating with the other end of the humerus are the two bones of the forearm, called the radius and the ulna. The radius and ulna permit rotation of the forearm. The "funny bone" is located at the end of the ulna, next to the humerus. The wrist is composed of eight small bones called the carpals. The arrangement of these bones permits the rotating movements of the wrist. The palm of the hand consists of five bones, known as the metacarpals, each of which articulates with a bone of the finger, called a phalanx. Each finger has three phalanges, with the exception of the thumb, which has two.

The pattern of bones in the leg and foot is similar to that in the arm and hand. The upper leg bone, called the femur, articulates with the pelvic girdle. The two lower leg bones are the tibia (shinbone) and fibula, corresponding to the radius and ulna of the arm, respectively. These two bones are responsible for rotation of the lower leg. Ventral to the joint between the upper and lower leg bones is another bone, the patella or knee cap, which serves as a point of muscle attachment for upper and lower leg muscles. This bone has no counterpart in the arm. The ankle contains seven irregularly shaped bones, the tarsals, corresponding to the carpals of the wrist. The foot proper contains five metatarsals, corresponding to the metacarpals of the hand, and the bones in the toes are the phalanges, two in the big toe and three in each of the others.

6.7 Articulations

Articulations (joints) are the structures where bones connect. There are three main classes of articulations based on the amount of motion they allow:

Synarthroses - A synarthrosis is an immovable joint (fibrous joint). One example is a suture. The parietal bones are locked together by a **sagittal suture**. The frontal bone is united to each of the parietal bones by a **coronal suture**.

Amphiarthroses - An amphiarthrosis is a joint permitting slight mobility. It is also known as a cartilaginous joint. One example is the symphysis pubis, where the two os coxa bones join anteriorly.

Diarthroses - A diarthrosis allows free mobility. It is also called a synovial joint. There are six subclasses within this main class:

Ball and Socket - The head of one bone (e.g., femur) fits into a shallow depression (e.g., glenoid fossa of the scapula). Motion occurs here in three different planes.

Hinge - One example is the knee joint. Another is the elbow joint.

Pivot - The ring of one bone rotates around the process of another. The atlas pivots on the axis.

Gliding - Bones can slide over each other. Examples occur among the carpal and tarsal bones.

Saddle - The bones have a saddle shape. Examples occur between the carpals and metacarpals.

Condyloid - An oval-shaped condyle of one bone fits into an elliptical shape of another. The metacarpals join the phalanges.

Problem Solving Example:

Q What is meant by a joint? What different types of joints are there?

A The point of junction between two bones is called a joint. Some joints, such as those between the bones of the skull, are immovable and extremely strong, owing to an intricate intermeshing of the edges of the bones. The truly movable joints of the skeleton are those that give the skeleton its importance in the total effector mechanism of locomotion. Some are ball-and-socket joints, such as the joint where the femur joins the pelvis, or where the humerus joins the pectoral girdle. These joints allow free movement in several directions. Both the pelvis and the pectoral girdle contain rounded, concave depressions to accommodate the rounded convex heads of the femur and humerus, respectively. Hinge joints, such as that of the human knee, permit movement in one direction only. The pivot joints at the wrists and ankles allow freedom of movement intermediate between that of the hinge and the ball and socket types.

The different bones of a joint are held together by connective tissue strands called ligaments. Skeletal muscles, attached to the bones by means of another type of connective tissue strand known as a tendon, produce their effects by bending the skeleton at the movable joints. The ends of each bone at a movable joint are covered with a layer of smooth cartilage. These bearing surfaces are completely enclosed in a liquid-tight capsule, called the bursa.

The joint cavity is filled with a liquid lubricant, called the synovial fluid, which is secreted by the synovial membrane lining the cavity. (Refer to the diagrams below.) During youth and early maturity, the lubricant is replaced as needed, but in middle and old age, the supply is often decreased, resulting in joint stiffness and difficulty of movement.

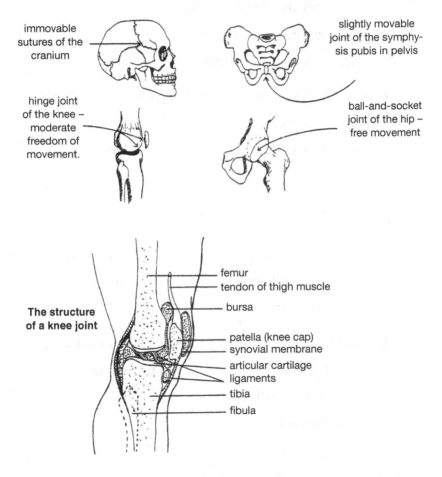

Diagrams illustrating the types of joints found in the human body

Quiz: The Skeletal System

1. When bone formation takes place in preexisting cartilage, it is called

    (A) intramembranous bone formation.

    (B) primary ossification.

    (C) endochondral ossification.

    (D) subchondral ossification.

    (E) metaplastic ossification.

2. Which of the following is part of the appendicular skeleton?

    (A) Humerus   (D) Sternum

    (B) Vertebrae   (E) Skull

    (C) Ribs

3. Knee and elbow joints are examples of bone articulations known as

    (A) synarthroses.   (D) diarthroses.

    (B) synchondroses.   (E) synovioses.

    (C) amphiarthroses.

4. A band of connective tissue that binds bone to bone is known as a

    (A) tendon.   (D) choroid plexus.

    (B) chorda tendinea.   (E) menisci.

    (C) ligament.

5. Compact bone would most likely be found

    (A) directly underneath the periosteum.

    (B) in the medullary cavity of a long bone.

    (C) on either side of the epiphyseal line of adult bone.

    (D) in the secondary ossification centers of fetal bone.

    (E) within cancellous bone.

6. In humans, the large bone extending from the hip to the knee is called the

    (A) tibia.   (D) humerus.

    (B) fibula.   (E) femur.

    (C) patella.

7. The proximal epiphyseal plate of a human humerus would be closest to which of the following?

    (A) The ulna

    (B) The insertion of the triceps brachii

    (C) The scapula

    (D) The insertion of the biceps brachii

    (E) The clavicle

8. Which of the following is part of a human's axial skeleton?

    (A) Clavicle   (D) Rib

    (B) Fibula   (E) Scapula

    (C) Humerus

9. Name the bone that does not articulate with the humerus.

    (A) Clavicle   (D) Shoulder blade

    (B) Radius   (E) Ulna

    (C) Scapula

10. The shaft of a long bone is properly known as the

    (A) diaphysis.

    (B) epiphysis.

    (C) amphiarthrosis.

    (D) symphysis.

    (E) diathesis.

ANSWER KEY

1.	(C)	6.	(E)
2.	(A)	7.	(C)
3.	(D)	8.	(D)
4.	(C)	9.	(A)
5.	(A)	10.	(A)

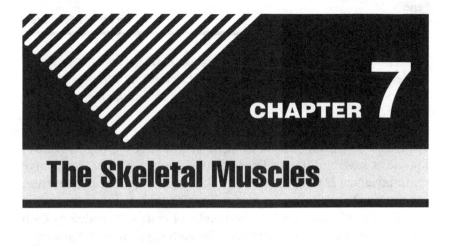

CHAPTER 7

The Skeletal Muscles

7.1 Functions

Skeletal muscles carry out several important body functions.

Movement - Skeletal muscles attach to the bones. As a muscle contracts, it pulls on a bone (or bones) to produce movement. For example, the hamstring muscles are found in the posterior thigh. As each contracts, it pulls the calf toward the thigh, producing flexion (bending) of the calf. As it contracts, a muscle pulls an **insertion bone** (movable end) toward an **origin bone** (fixed end). In this example, the tibia represents the insertion bone and the femur represents the origin bone.

Heat Production - Numerous chemical reactions in muscle cells liberate heat. This heat contributes to the maintenance of body temperature.

Posture - Some skeletal muscles pull on the vertebral column and other parts of the skeleton, helping to maintain an upright stance and posture of the body.

7.2 Structure of a Skeletal Muscle

There are more than 600 skeletal muscles in the human body. Each one has the same basic structure at several levels of organization: organ (the muscle), tissue (striated, skeletal), cell (fiber), organelles (e.g., mitochondria and myofibrils), and molecules (e.g., water, actin, myosin).

As an organ, a skeletal muscle consists of several tissue types. Skeletal muscle **fibers** are long, thread-like cells that compose skeletal (striated) tissue. These cells have the ability to shorten their length or contract.

Dense fibrous connective tissue (fascia) weaves through a skeletal muscle at several different levels. The **epimysium** is the connective tissue layer that envelopes the entire skeletal muscle. The **perimysium** is a continuation of this outer fascia, dividing the interior of the muscle into bundles of muscle cells. The bundle of cells surrounded by each perimysium is called a fasciculus. The **endomysium** is a connective tissue layer surrounding each muscle fiber.

The interior of a muscle also contains the axons of motor neurons. Each axon signals a group of muscle fibers. This association (one neuron, group of muscle fibers) is called a **motor unit**.

Muscles also contain an abundant supply of blood vessels. The blood delivers glucose and other nutrients, along with oxygen, that are needed for cell metabolism. There are also fat deposits in muscles that store energy.

Muscle cells contain many organelles common to most cells (i.e., mitochondria). **Myofibrils** are organelles that establish the contractile ability of muscle cells. Each myofibril is a linear succession of box-like units called **sarcomeres**. Each sarcomere contains the contractile proteins (myofilaments) **actin** and **myosin**. The myosin is the thicker central protein. The actin is the thinner protein at each end of the sarcomere.

Actin and myosin are organized in each sarcomere in the following regions:

A Band - Actin and myosin

H Zone - Myosin only, within the A band

I Band - Actin only

Z Line - Boundary of the sarcomere where actin molecules are attached at each end

Problem Solving Example:

 The most widely accepted theory of muscle contraction is the sliding filament theory. What is the major point of this theory?

A The major premise of the sliding filament theory is that muscle contraction occurs as the result of the sliding of the thick and thin filaments past one another; the lengths of the individual filaments remain unchanged. Thus, the width of the A band remains constant, corresponding to the constant length of the thick filaments. The I band narrows as the thin filaments approach the center of the sarcomere. As the thin filaments move past the thick filaments, the width of the H zone between the ends of the thin filaments becomes smaller and may disappear altogether when the thin filaments meet at the center of the sarcomere. With further shortening, new banding patterns appear as thin filaments from opposite ends of the sarcomere begin to overlap. The shortening of the sarcomeres in a myofibril is the direct cause of the shortening of the whole muscle.

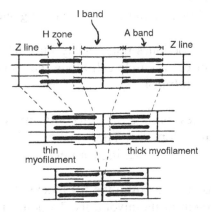

Changes in banding pattern resulting from the movements of thick and thin filaments past each other during contraction

The question arises as to which structures actually produce the sliding of the filaments. The answer is the myosin crossbridges. These crossbridges are actually part of the myosin molecules that compose the thick filaments. The bridges swivel in an arc around their fixed positions on the surface of the thick filaments, much like the oars of a boat. When bound to the actin filaments, the movement of the crossbridges causes the sliding of the thick and thin filaments past each other. Since one movement of a crossbridge will produce only a small displacement of the filaments relative to each other, the crossbridges must undergo many repeated cycles of movement during contraction.

7.3 Mechanism of a Muscle Contraction

A skeletal muscle contracts by the following series of steps:

1. A motor nerve signals the muscle. Some of the neurons in the nerve develop electrical impulses that signal some fibers in the muscle. Each axon secretes a **neurotransmitter** (chemical signal) called **acetylcholine** at the **synapse** (motor end plate) between the neuron and some muscle fibers. This signal excites each signaled muscle cell.

2. An electrical signal spreads out along the **sarcolemma** (cell membrane) of each muscle cell that is signaled.

3. This signal continues transversely into the **sarcoplasm** (cytoplasm) of each muscle cell along the membranes of the **T (transverse) tubules**.

4. The T tubules join the **SR (sarcoplasmic reticulum)** in the sarcoplasm (cytoplasm). The signal spreads from the T tubules to this tubular SR, releasing **Ca ions**.

5. The release of Ca^{+2} from the SR blocks the action of **troponin**, a protein in the myofibrils. Troponin normally inhibits the interaction of actin and myosin, contractile proteins in the sarcomeres of the myofibrils.

6. With troponin inhibited, actin and myosin can interact. Cross-bridges on the myosin slide the actin molecules toward the center of the sarcomere. As the actin molecules are attached to the Z lines, boundaries of the sarcomeres, this shortens the sarcomeres according to the **sliding filament theory**. The actin molecules slide between the central myosin molecules.

7. **Hydrolysis** of **ATP** in the cells, into ADP and phosphate, releases energy to drive the sliding of the filaments (actin and myosin). ATP is rebuilt from an energy-storage compound, creatine phosphate.

8. If enough sarcomeres shorten, myofibrils shorten. If enough myofibrils shorten, the fibers (cells) shorten. If enough fibers shorten, the muscle shortens or contracts.

Each muscle responds by an **all-or-none** law. If stimulated sufficiently, it contracts fully. The force of contraction from an entire muscle depends on the percentage of cells that are active, each cell responding by all-or-none.

Problem Solving Example:

 What are the properties of actin and myosin that produce the cyclic activity of the crossbridges responsible for contraction?

 Myosin, the larger of the two molecules, is shaped like a lollipop (see figure on the next page). The myosin molecules are arranged within the thick filaments so that they are oriented tail-to-tail in the two halves of the filament; the globular ends extend to the sides, forming the crossbridges that bind to the reactive site on the actin molecule. Actin is a globular-shaped molecule having a reactive site on its surface that is able to combine with myosin. These globular proteins are arranged in two chains that are helically intertwined to form the thin myofilaments (see figure on the next page).

The globular end of the myosin molecule, in addition to being a binding site for the actin molecule, contains a separate binding site for

ATP. This active site has ATPase activity, and the reaction that is catalyzed is the hydrolysis of ATP.

$$H_2O + ATP \longrightarrow ADP + P_i$$

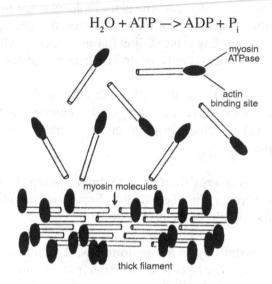

Aggregation of myosin molecules to form thick filaments, with the globular heads of the myosin molecules forming the crossbridges

Structure of thin myofilament composed of two helical chains of globular actin monomers

However, myosin alone has a very low ATPase activity. It appears that an allosteric change occurs in the active site of myosin ATPase when the myosin crossbridge combines with actin in the thin filaments, considerably increasing the ATPase activity. The energy that is released from the splitting of ATP produces crossbridge movement by an as yet unknown mechanism. It is believed that the oscillatory movements of myosin crossbridges produce the relative movement of thick and thin filaments, resulting ultimately in the shortening of a muscle fiber (see figure below).

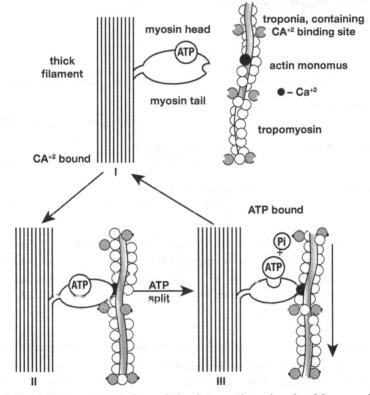

Schematic representation of the interactions involved in muscle contractions

Since many cycles of activity are needed to produce the degree of shortening observed during muscle contraction, the myosin bridge must be able to detach from the actin and then rebind again. To accomplish this, ATP binds to the myosin in the crossbridge, forming what is known as a low energy complex. The low energy complex has only a weak affinity for actin; the actin-myosin bond is broken, allowing the crossbridges to dissociate from actin. Shortly after this event, a conformational change occurs in the myosin—ATP complex, and a high energy complex is formed. The high energy complex has a very high affinity for actin, and the crossbridges are able to rebind to the actin. In this manner, the crossbridges are able to bind and dissociate from actin in a cycle of coordinated actions. This cycle may be summarized in the following sequence of events:

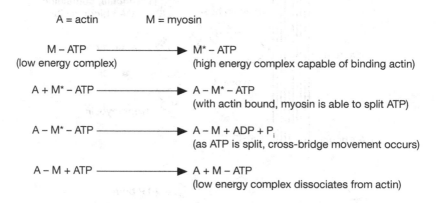

A = actin   M = myosin

M – ATP ──────────────▶ M* – ATP
(low energy complex)   (high energy complex capable of binding actin)

A + M* – ATP ──────────▶ A – M* – ATP
                         (with actin bound, myosin is able to split ATP)

A – M* – ATP ──────────▶ A – M + ADP + P_i
                         (as ATP is split, cross-bridge movement occurs)

A – M + ATP ───────────▶ A + M – ATP
                         (low energy complex dissociates from actin)

At the molecular level, we can identify two specific roles for ATP: 1) to provide energy for movement of the crossbridge, and 2) to dissociate actin from the myosin crossbridges during the contraction cycle of the bridges. ATP is also needed to restore Ca^{+2} in the sarcoplasmic reticulum following contraction.

Two regulatory proteins, troponin and tropomyosin, are associated with actin. During nervous stimulation of a muscle, there is an increase in free intracellular calcium ions: calcium diffuses in from the terminal cisternae and from the extracellular fluid of the T tubules. Calcium binds to troponin, which causes tropomyosin to shift its position along the actin helix. This exposes the binding site on actin for myosin.

7.4   Patterns of a Muscle Contraction

There are several patterns of contraction of a skeletal muscle.

Tonus - Some motor units in a muscle are usually active when a muscle is not contracting enough to produce movement. The muscle remains taut by this tonic response. Tonus (muscle tone) of some muscles maintains posture.

Problem Solving Examples:

 What is meant by the term "tonus"?

 The term tonus refers to the state of sustained partial contraction present in skeletal muscles as long as the nerves to the muscle are intact. Unlike skeletal muscle, cardiac and smooth muscles exhibit tonus even after their nerves are cut. Tonus is a mild state of tetanus (a sustained maximum contraction). It is present at all times and involves only a small fraction of the fibers of a muscle at any one time. It is believed that the individual fibers contract in turn, working in relays, so that each fiber has a chance to recover completely while other fibers are contracting before it is called upon to contract again. A muscle under slight tension can react more rapidly and contract more strongly than one that is completely relaxed because of changes in the elastic component in the latter.

Isometric/Isotonic - By isometric response, a muscle does not contract enough to produce motion (isometric = equal length). It stabilizes a body part. For example, muscles in the shoulder act isometrically if the arms push against an immovable wall. By isotonic response, a muscle does shorten and produces motion.

 Differentiate between an isometric and an isotonic contraction.

Contraction refers to the active process of generating a force in a muscle. The force exerted by a contracting muscle on an object is known as the muscle tension, and the force exerted on a muscle by the weight of an object is known as the load. When a muscle shortens and lifts a load, the muscle contraction is said to be isotonic, since the load remains constant throughout the period of shortening.

When a load is greater than the muscle tension, shortening is prevented, and muscle length remains constant. Likewise, when a load is supported in a fixed position by the tension of the muscle, the muscle length remains constant. This development of muscle tension at a constant muscle length is said to be an isometric contraction. The internal physiochemical events are the same in both isotonic and isometric contraction. Movement of the limbs involves isotonic contractions, whereas maintaining one's posture requires isometric contractions.

Isotonic responses can be graphed as several patterns (see figure on the next page).

Simple Twitch - Quick, jerky contraction to a single stimulus.

Summation - The addition of simple twitches from repeated stimulation of a muscle—the twitches add together (summate) toward a more powerful, unified response. This often occurs when the nervous system signals a muscle at a faster rate, causing the twitches to merge.

Tetanus - The powerful, sustained contraction of a muscle from the summation of simple twitches. Isotonic responses of skeletal muscles in the body are usually tetanic.

Problem Solving Example:

Q The property of skeletal muscle contraction in which the mechanical response to one or more successive stimuli is added to the first is known as summation. What is the underlying explanation of this phenomenon?

A A possible explanation of this phenomenon, based on the role of calcium in excitation-contraction coupling, is that the amount of calcium released from the sarcoplasmic reticulum during a single action potential is sufficient to inhibit only some of the troponin-tropomyosin in the muscle. Multiple stimulation would then release more calcium so that more troponin-tropomyosin would be inhibited, allowing for further contraction. However, the truth is that more than enough calcium is released by the first action potential to inhibit all the troponin-tropomyosin, so this proposal must be discarded.

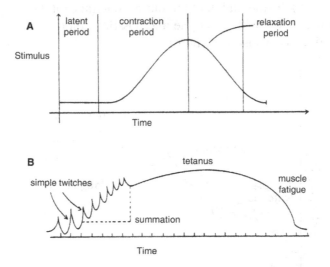

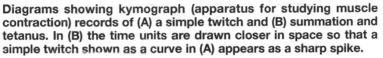

Diagrams showing kymograph (apparatus for studying muscle contraction) records of (A) a simple twitch and (B) summation and tetanus. In (B) the time units are drawn closer in space so that a simple twitch shown as a curve in (A) appears as a sharp spike.

The explanation of summation involves the passive elastic properties of the muscle. Tension is transmitted from the crossbridges through the thick and thin filaments, across the Z lines, and eventually through the extracellular connective tissue and the tendons to the bone. All these structures have a certain amount of elasticity, analogous to a spring that is placed between the contractile components of the muscle and the external object. In the muscle, the contractile elements in their fully active state begin to stretch the passive elastic structures immediately following calcium release. Only when the elastic structures are all taut can increasing contraction by the muscle occur. Summation occurs because a second stimulus is given, very close in time to the first, while the elastic structures are still a bit taut and not yet slack. Under this condition, the active state of the contractile proteins is maintained, and the result is contractions that are stronger than any single simple twitch. Should sustained stimulation occur, the elastic elements would never have time to relax at all, and it is at this point that maximal force by the muscle fibers is attained; the individual contractions are indistinguishably fused into a single sustained contraction known as tetanus (see figure below). If stimulation of the muscle continues at this frequency, the ultimate result will be fatigue and possibly complete cessation of activity due to exhaustion of nutrients.

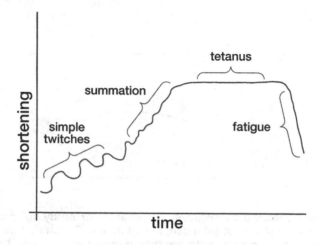

Graph of simple twitches, summation, tetanus, and fatigue

It is not surprising to note that cardiac muscle has an extremely long refractory period, allowing the elastic components to relax and thus avoiding tetanus, which would result in death due to loss of pumping action of the heart.

Fatigue - The muscle cannot respond when stimulated, as it is exhausted of nutrients and accumulates waste products. The muscle can be depleted of glucose, a source of energy. Lactic acid is a waste product that builds up in muscle cells during anaerobic conditions, which means an absence of oxygen. This occurs when an overworked muscle does not receive oxygen rapidly enough to meet its metabolic needs.

Problem Solving Example:

Q What is meant by the term muscle fatigue?

A A muscle that has contracted several times, exhausting its stored supply of organic phosphates and glycogen, will accumulate lactic acid. It is unable to contract any longer and is said to be "fatigued." Fatigue is primarily induced by this accumulation of lactic acid, which correlates closely with the depletion of the muscle stores of glycogen. Fatigue, however, may actually be felt by the individual before the muscle reaches the exhausted condition.

The spot most susceptible to fatigue can be demonstrated experimentally. A muscle and its attached nerve can be dissected out and the nerve stimulated repeatedly by electric shock until the muscle no longer contracts. If the muscle is then stimulated directly by placing electrodes on the muscle tissue, it will contract. With the proper device for detecting the passage of nerve impulses, it can be shown that upon fatigue, the nerve leading to the muscle is not fatigued, but remains capable of conduction. Thus, since the nerve is still conducting impulses and the muscle is still capable of contracting, the point of fatigue must be at the junction between the nerve and the muscle, where nerve impulses initiate muscle contraction. Fatigue is then due in part to an accumulation of lactic acid, in part to depletion of stored energy reserves, and in part to breakdown in neuromuscular junction transmission.

In contrast to true muscle fatigue, psychological fatigue may cause an individual to stop exercising even though his or her muscles are not depleted of ATP and are still able to contract. An athlete's performance depends not only upon the physical state of his or her muscles but also upon his or her will to perform.

7.5 Motions

Skeletal muscles attach to bones by tendons. At movable joints (diarthroses), a contracting muscle can pull on a bone (or bones) to produce one of the following motions (actions):

Flexion - Bending, decreasing the angle at a joint

Extension - Straightening out, increasing the angle at a joint

Abduction - Moving a limb away from the midline of the body

Adduction - Moving a limb toward the midline of the body

Rotation - Pivoting a structure—the atlas (C1) and skull can rotate on the axis (C2). A special case of rotation is pronation and supination. Through **pronation**, the palm is turned posteriorly (radius crosses over the ulna). Through **supination**, it is turned to an anterior position (radius and ulna become parallel).

Dorsiflexion - The toes are lifted as the body is supported on the heels.

Plantar Flexion - The heels are lifted and the body is supported on the toes.

Inversion - The toes are pointed medially.

Eversion - The toes are pointed laterally.

To produce a given body motion, muscles work in groups. Each member has a specific role. In forearm flexion, for example, the biceps brachii is the **prime mover**. It contracts and is mainly responsible for the action. The triceps brachii is the **antagonist**. It could oppose the prime mover, but relaxes. Other muscles, called **synergists**, contract to support the action of the prime mover. These roles can be applied to any muscle group producing an action.

Problem Solving Example:

What is meant by an antagonistic muscle? Give examples.

Muscles can exert a pull but not a push. For this reason, muscles are typically arranged in antagonistic pairs: one pulls a bone in one direction and the other pulls it in the opposite direction. The biceps, for example, bends or flexes the arm and is termed a flexor. Its antagonist, the triceps, straightens or extends the arm and is termed an extensor (see accompanying figure). Such pairs of opposing extensors and flexors are found at the wrist, ankle, and knee, as well as at other joints. When either the flexor or the extensor contracts, its antagonistic muscle must relax to permit the bone to move. The proper coordination of nerve impulses is necessary for antagonistic pairs to function properly.

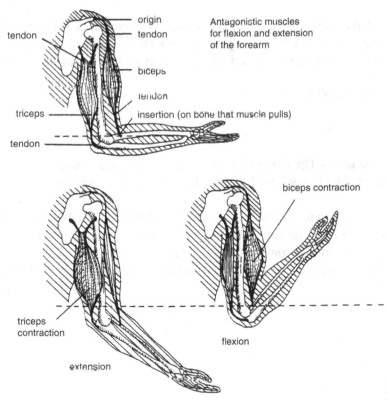

Other antagonistic pairs of muscles are adductors and abductors, which move parts of the body toward or away from the central axis of the body, respectively; levators and depressors raise or lower parts of the body; and while pronators rotate parts of the body downward and backward, supinators rotate them upward and forward.

7.6   Naming of Skeletal Muscles

The skeletal muscles are named according to the following characteristics. Often two or more of these are applied to the name of the muscle. Here are a few examples:

Location - The tibialis anterior is in front of the shinbone.

Number of Attachments - The biceps brachii has two origins (fixed ends of attachments). The triceps brachii has three origins.

Direction of Fibers - The fibers of the rectus abdominis muscles range straight (rectus = straight) or parallel to the long axis of the body. The fibers of the external oblique range at an angle (oblique) to this axis.

Shape/Size - The deltoid has the shape of a triangle (delta = triangle). The gluteus maximus of the buttocks is larger compared to the gluteus minimus.

Action - The extensor muscles in the forearm straighten out the fingers. The flexor muscles in the forearm bend the fingers.

A muscle name can reveal two characteristics. The biceps brachii and triceps brachii are found in the upper arm (brachion = arm). The rectus abdominis composes part of the abdominal wall. The external oblique is superficial compared to the internal oblique of the abdominal wall.

7.7   Skeletal Muscles - Body Regions

Some major superficial (surface) skeletal muscles throughout the regions of the body are:

Buccinator - In the cheek—it contracts to compress the cheeks.

Masseter - Inserting on the posterior region on the mandible—it raises the mandible, contributing to mastication (chewing).

Temporalis - Fan-shaped muscle covering the temporal bone—it supplements (synergistic) the action of the masseter.

Orbicularis Oculi - Circular muscle around the anterior margin of the orbit (eye socket)—it closes the eye.

Orbicularis Oris - Circular muscle around the anterior margin of the mouth—it contracts to pucker the lips.

Sternocleidomastoid - Diagonal muscle on each side of the neck, ranging from sternum and clavicle (origins) to the mastoid process of the temporal bone (insertion)—when both contract, the head is flexed toward the chest.

Deltoid - Bulging muscle that covers each shoulder—it abducts the upper arm.

Biceps Brachii - Major muscle of the anterior upper arm—it flexes the forearm.

Triceps Brachii - Major muscle of the posterior upper arm—it extends the forearm.

Pectoralis Major - Major chest muscle—it adducts the upper arm with some medial rotation.

Rectus Abdominis - Midline, segmented muscle of the abdominal wall—it flexes the trunk.

External Oblique - Located on each side of the rectus abdominis—each one bends the trunk to that side of the body.

Trapezius - Large, diamond-shaped muscle of the upper back—it extends the head and works to shrug the shoulders.

Latissimus Dorsi - Wide muscle of the lower back—it extends and adducts the upper arm.

Gluteus Maximus - The largest muscle of the buttocks—it extends the thigh.

Rectus Femoris - Located along the front of the femur—it flexes the thigh. It combines with three other thigh muscles (**vastus lateralis, vastus intermedius, vastus medialis**) to form the **quadriceps** muscle. They act to extend the calf.

Sartorius - Long, ribbon-like muscle ranging over the front of the thigh—it is used to cross the legs.

Biceps Femoris and Semitendinosus - The lateral and medial hamstring muscles respectively, located on the posterior thigh—they flex the calf.

Tibialis Anterior - Along the front of the tibia—it produces dorsiflexion.

Gastrocnemius - The bulging posterior calf muscle—it produces plantar flexion.

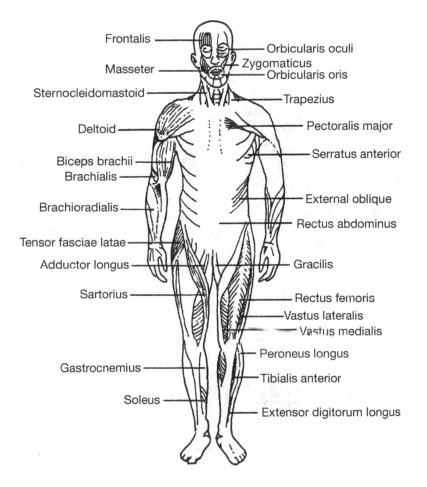

Frontalis

Masseter

Sternocleidomastoid

Deltoid

Biceps brachii
Brachialis

Brachioradialis

Tensor fasciae latae

Adductor longus

Sartorius

Gastrocnemius

Soleus

Orbicularis oculi
Zygomaticus
Orbicularis oris

Trapezius

Pectoralis major

Serratus anterior

External oblique

Rectus abdominus

Gracilis

Rectus femoris
Vastus lateralis
Vastus medialis

Peroneus longus

Tibialis anterior

Extensor digitorum longus

Superficial muscles — anterior

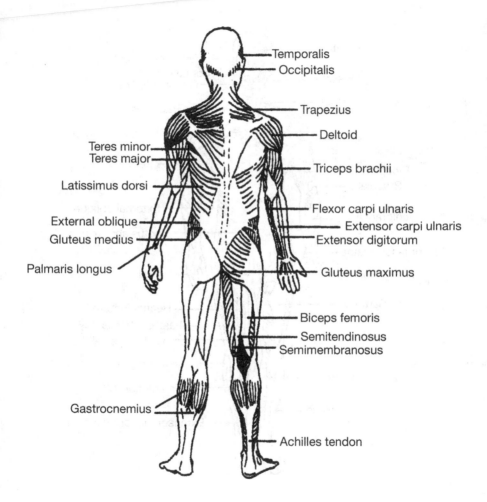

- Temporalis
- Occipitalis
- Trapezius
- Deltoid
- Teres minor
- Teres major
- Triceps brachii
- Latissimus dorsi
- Flexor carpi ulnaris
- External oblique
- Extensor carpi ulnaris
- Gluteus medius
- Extensor digitorum
- Palmaris longus
- Gluteus maximus
- Biceps femoris
- Semitendinosus
- Semimembranosus
- Gastrocnemius
- Achilles tendon

Superficial muscles—posterior

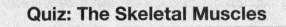

Quiz: The Skeletal Muscles

1. When a muscle contracts, tension develops because of

    (A) interaction between the actin and myosin filaments.

    (B) the overlapping arrangement of the actin and myosin filaments.

    (C) a slackening within the connective tissue elements.

    (D) the length-tension relationship.

    (E) the shortening of the actin filament.

2. Which of the following ions or molecules is bound to myosin when the muscle fiber is not contracting (at rest)?

    (A) ATP

    (B) Ca^{+2}

    (C) Na^+

    (D) ADP

    (E) $ADP + P_i$

3. Which of the following gives the correct composition of the thin myofilaments that are attached to the Z lines of a sarcomere?

    (A) Actin, myosin, troponin

    (B) Myosin, tropomyosin, troponin

    (C) Actin, troponin, tropomyosin

    (D) Myosin, actin, tropomyosin

    (E) Tropomyosin, myosin, troponin

4. During muscle contraction, the Ca^{+2} that is released combines with

    (A) troponin.   (D) fibrinogen.

    (B) actomyosin.   (E) None of the above.

    (C) tropomyosin.

5. Muscles pull on bones from their

    (A) antagonists to prime movers.

    (B) insertions to origins.

    (C) origins to insertions.

    (D) prime movers to synergists.

    (E) synergists to antagonists.

6. The protein that also serves as an enzyme that breaks down
    $ATP \rightarrow ADP = P_i$ during muscle contraction is

    (A) tropomyosin.   (D) troponin.

    (B) fibrinogen.   (E) regulator protein.

    (C) actomyosin.

7. The basic contractile unit in striated muscle is

    (A) the muscle fiber.   (D) the myofilament.

    (B) the myofibril.   (E) the thin filaments.

    (C) the sarcomere.

8. All of the following occurs as muscles contract EXCEPT

    (A) Z bands come closer.

    (B) H zones stay the same.

    (C) A bands stay the same.

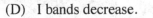
(D)   I bands decrease.

(E)   thick and thin filaments slide past each other.

9.   Striated (skeletal) muscle fibers exhibit

(A)   few mitochondria.

(B)   alternating A bands and I bands in a transverse pattern.

(C)   only one nucleus.

(D)   no orderly arrangement.

(E)   All of the above.

10.   Muscle fatigue is due, in part, to the accumulation of

(A)   lactic acid.

(B)   citric acid.

(C)   pyruvic acid.

(D)   ACTH.

(E)   ATP.

ANSWER KEY

1.	(A)	6.	(D)
2.	(A)	7.	(C)
3.	(C)	8.	(B)
4.	(A)	9.	(B)
5.	(B)	10.	(A)

CHAPTER 8

The Nervous System

8.1 Divisions of the Nervous System

The nervous system is a major communication network that sends signals throughout the body. It consists of two major divisions. The two divisions are connected and work together.

Central Nervous System (CNS) - This division consists of the **brain** and **spinal cord**. The brain is contained within the cranium. The spinal cord is found within the vertebral column, extending from the base of the skull to the first lumbar vertebra.

Peripheral Nervous System (PNS) - This division consists of 12 pairs of **cranial nerves** and 31 pairs of **spinal nerves**. They are continuous with the brain and spinal cord, respectively. However, just as branches are connected to the trunk of a tree, the cranial nerves and spinal nerves are located outside the central branch.

The **autonomic nervous system** is a subdivision of the PNS. It controls motor functions of the internal organs (viscera). It has two branches, the sympathetic and parasympathetic. These two branches have opposing effects on the activity of an organ. All remaining peripheral control is carried out by the **somatic nervous system**, the other branch of the PNS.

8.2   Neuron/Glial Cell

The **neuron** is the cell of the nervous system that sends impulses (see figure on the next page). **Glial cells** protect and provide support for the neurons. They also provide nourishment.

The neuron has the following regions and specializations:

Cell Body - Contains the nucleus and most of the cytoplasm.

Dendrite - This process sends the impulse toward the cell body. There may be one or many dendrites per cell. Some neurons lack dendrites.

Axon - This process sends the impulse away from the cell body. There is only one axon per neuron. It is also called the nerve fiber.

Myelin Sheath - This is a white, fatty covering around the axon. It is produced in the PNS by a type of glial cell, the **Schwann cell**, that wraps around the axon. It deposits the myelin around the axon in a series of circular layers. Masses of axons that are myelinated in the nervous system compose the white matter. Unmyelinated axons, plus dendrites and cell bodies, compose the gray matter.

Nodes of Ranvier - These are the gaps between Schwann cells along the axon. Where these cells are absent, there are also gaps in the myelin covering the axon, the nodes.

Neurilemma - This is a thin covering along the axon that is external to the myelin when present. It promotes the regeneration of the axon.

There are several kinds of neurons:

Sensory (Afferent) - This neuron sends signals toward the CNS. It has long dendrites and a short axon.

Motor (Efferent) - This neuron is found in nerves and sends signals away from the CNS. It has short dendrites or the dendrites may be absent. The axon is long.

Interneuron - This cell is found between sensory and motor neurons. It is contained within the CNS.

The several kinds of neurons work together to establish circuits throughout the body. They are separated by junctions between them called **synapses**. For example, a painful stimulus is conducted to the CNS by sensory neurons. A response to this, such as pulling the arm away from the stimulus, is controlled by motor neurons. Interneurons between the sensory and motor neurons complete the circuit needed for this action.

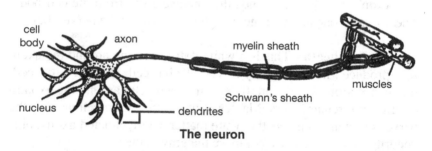

cell body | axon | myelin sheath | muscles | Schwann's sheath | nucleus | dendrites

The neuron

Problem Solving Example:

Q What is the structure of a typical neuron?

A Many types of neurons are present in humans (see figure on the next page). Nevertheless, often three parts of a neuron can be distinguished: a cell body, an axon, and a group of processes called dendrites.

Dendrites are usually rather short and numerous extensions from the cell body. They frequently branch profusely, and their many short terminals may give them a spiny appearance. When stained, they ordinarily show many dark granules. There is usually only one axon per neuron (very rarely two), and it is frequently longer than the dendrites.

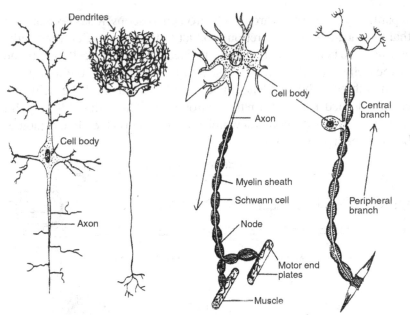

A variety of neuron types in human beings

It may branch extensively, but unlike dendrites, it does not have a spiny appearance and does not show dark granules when stained. The most fundamental distinction between dendrites and axons is that dendrites receive excitation from other cells, whereas axons generally do not, and that axons can stimulate other cells, whereas dendrites cannot. Thus, dendrites carry information to the cell body, while axons carry information away from the cell body.

Axons may be several feet long in some neurons. A bundle of many axons wrapped together by a sheath of connective tissue is what is commonly called a nerve. Each vertebrate axon is usually enveloped in a myelin sheath formed by special cells, the Schwann cells, that almost completely encircle the axon. Schwann cells play a role in the nutrition of the axons, and provide a conduit within which damaged axons can grow from the cell body back to their original position. The myelin sheath is interrupted at regular intervals; the interruptions are called nodes of Ranvier. At these nodes, the myelin sheath disappears. The myelin functions in speeding up the transmission of impulses in the axon it envelopes. It is crucial to note that the myelin sheath is not a separate layer by itself. Through electron microscopy, it has been proven that the sheath is not a secretion product of the axon or Schwann cells, as was once believed, but a tightly packed spiral of the cell membrane of the Schwann cells. Thus, the sheath is composed of the lipid from the membrane's bilayer. The nucleus and cytoplasm of the Schwann cell are pushed aside to form the neurolemma. The nodes in the myelin sheath are simply the points at which one Schwann cell ends and another begins (see figure below).

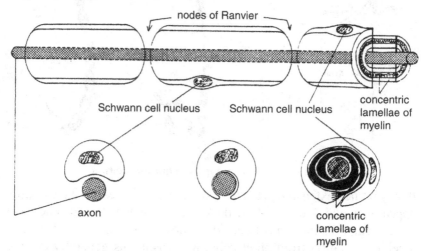

Sheath cells on a neuron. (upper) Dissection of a myelinated nerve fiber. (lower) Envelopment of axis cylinder by a sheath cell.

The neuronal cell body, or perikaryon, contains the nucleus and cytoplasmic organelles distributed around the nucleus. The perikaryon has well-developed endoplasmic reticulum and Golgi apparatus for manufacturing all the substances needed for the maintenance and functioning of the axon and dendrites.

8.2.1 Nerve Impulse

The nerve impulse, called the **action potential**, is electrical in nature. It develops by the following events.

1. The **resting membrane potential** occurs in a neuron when it is not firing an impulse. The cell is positive extracellularly and

negative intracellularly. It is positive on the outside due to a higher concentration of sodium ions.

2. When stimulated, the cell membrane becomes more permeable to sodium ions. These ions are positive. Some of these ions diffuse into the cell. This change travels point by point along the cell membrane, reversing the polarity of the cell (wave of depolarization). The electrical change (positive on the inside, negative on the outside) is called the action potential.

3. After the impulse has passed along the neuron, the normal polarity of the cell is restored. The membrane becomes more permeable to potassium ions, which are higher in concentration intracellularly. They diffuse to the outside, point by point, along the cell membrane. This reestablishes the resting membrane potential.

Each time the neuron fires an impulse, some sodium diffuses into the cell, and some potassium ions diffuse to the outside. The sodium-potassium pump, working by active transport within the cell membrane, is independent of the action potential. It keeps sodium high on the outside and potassium high on the inside. By this activity the neuron remains prepared to change electrically to fire impulses.

Along a neuron the impulse travels from dendrite(s) to cell body to axon (**one-way conduction**).

Neurons that send impulses most rapidly are large and myelinated with nodes. Myelin prevents the diffusion of sodium and potassium ions. Therefore, the impulse jumps from node to node, where the myelin is absent, speeding up impulse transmission.

Problem Solving Examples:

What is a resting potential? Describe the chemical mechanism responsible for the resting potential. How can a resting potential be detected?

A There is a difference in electrical potential between the inside and the outside of all living cells. For example, the potential difference across the cell membrane of the neuron is measured to be about 60 millivolts, the inside being negative with respect to the outside. This potential difference is called the resting potential.

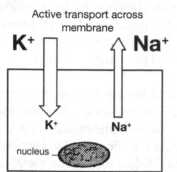

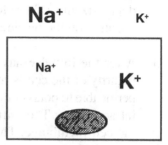

1. K⁺ ions are actively transported into the cell while Na⁺ ions are actively transported out of the cell.

2. K⁺ ions moving in and NA⁺ ions moving out lead to an accumulation of K⁺ ions in the cell and Na⁺ ions outside of the cell.

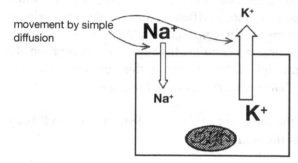

3. Permeability differences of K⁺ ions and Na⁺ ions across the membrane result in the net negative charge inside and the net positive charge outside the cell. This gives rise to the resting potential.

Diagrams showing the chemical mechanism responsible for the resting potential. Sizes of letters and arrows represent relative amounts present.

The chemical basis for the resting potential is as follows (refer to diagrams above). By active transport, an energy-requiring process that transfers substances across the cell membrane against their concentration gradients, the concentration of potassium (K^+) ions is kept higher inside the cell than outside. At the same time, there is a lower concentration of sodium (Na^+) ions in the cell interior than the exterior. Moreover, in the resting state the permeability of the cell membrane is different for K^+ and Na^+ ions. The membrane is more permeable to K^+

ions than to Na⁺ ions. Hence, K⁺ ions can move across the membrane by simple diffusion to the outside more easily than Na⁺ ions can move in to replace them. Because more positive charges (K⁺) leave the inside of the cell than are replenished (by Na⁺), there is a net negative charge on the inside and a net positive charge on the outside. An electrical potential is established across the membrane. This potential is the resting membrane potential.

We can measure the resting potential by placing one electrode, insulated except at the tip, inside the cell and a second electrode on the outside surface and connecting the two with a suitable recording device such as a sensitive galvanometer. The reading on the galvanometer should be approximately 60 millivolts if the cell tested is a neuron. (Different types of cells, such as skeletal and cardiac muscle cells, vary in their values of resting potential.) Note, however, that if both electrodes are placed on the outside surface of the cell, no potential difference between them is registered because all points on the outside are at equal potential. The same is true if both electrodes are placed on the inside surface of the plasma membrane.

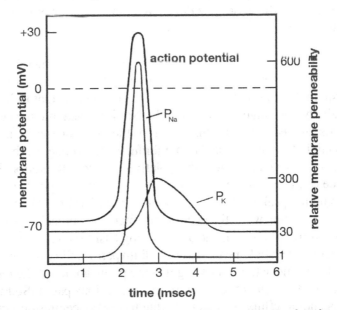

Changes in membrane permeability to sodium and potassium ions during an action potential

Q What is an action potential? Discuss the physical and electro-chemical changes during an action potential.

A We know that an unstimulated nerve cell exhibits a resting potential of about 60 millivolts across its membrane. An active pumping mechanism within the membrane causes the cell interior to accumulate a high concentration of K^+ ions and the exterior a high concentration of Na^+ ions. Since the resting membrane is 50 to 75 times more permeable to K^+ than to Na^+, more K^+ moves by simple diffusion out of the cell than Na^+ moves into the cell in the resting state, and hence a potential difference exists across the membrane. Diffusion moves ions down their concentration gradients, which were established by the active transport pump.

When a region of the axonal membrane is stimulated by a neurotransmitter, that region undergoes a set of electrochemical changes that constitutes an action potential. An action potential can be detected as a spike on a recording device, with a rising phase, a peak, and a falling phase, each corresponding to the characteristic flow of ions across the membrane of the axon. The duration of an action potential in a neuron is about 1 msec (.001 sec).

During an action potential, the permeability of the membrane to Na^+ and K^+ ions is markedly altered. Initially, the membrane permeability to Na^+ undergoes a thousandfold increase, whereas that to K^+ remains relatively unchanged. Consequently, Na^+ ions rush into the cell. If one inserts an electrode into this region of the axon, one will find that the potential at the inside of the membrane starts to rise, as the influx of positive (Na^+) ions reduces the negativity of the cell interior. Soon, the inside of the membrane registers a net positive charge. The positivity rises until a peak is reached at about + 40 millivolts. This phase of the action potential, when the membrane potential approaches or even rises above zero, is known as the depolarizing (rising) phase. At the peak of the action potential, the increased sodium permeability is rapidly turned off, and immediately following this the permeability of the membrane to K^+ suddenly increases (see figure on previous page). Sodium entry stops and an efflux of K^+ results due to the concentration gradient of K^+. The membrane potential starts to move toward zero, then drops below zero and finally restores the pre-excitation, or resting, state (at 60 mV). This phase of the action potential, when the membrane potential moves toward its resting level, is called the repolarizing (declining) phase. How depolarization is brought to a stop and repolarization is brought about is explained by a rapid shutting off of the increased sodium permeability (sodium inactivation).

8.2.2 Synaptic Transmission

The nature of the signal at the synapse is chemical. It develops by the following steps.

1. A neuron (presynaptic) develops an action potential.

2. The action potential triggers the release of **neurotransmitter** molecules (chemical signal) from the axonal end of this neuron. The neurotransmitter, such as acetylcholine (ACh), is stored in vesicles in the axon.

3. The neurotransmitter diffuses across the synapse from the presynaptic cell.

4. The neurotransmitter excites the next cell, located on the other side of the synapse (postsynaptic).

5. Sodium begins to diffuse into the postsynaptic cell, starting the development of its action potential.

6. The neurotransmitter is broken down or transported away from the synapse. The release of neurotransmitter molecules again is necessary for another signal across the synapse.

Problem Solving Example:

 What are the chemical and physical processes involved in transmission at the synapse?

 The nervous system is composed of discrete units, the neurons, yet it behaves like a continuous system of transmission

of impulses. For this to occur, there have to be functional connections between neurons. These connections are known as synapses. A
synapse is an anatomically specialized junction between two neurons
lying adjacent to each other where the electric activity in one neuron
(the presynaptic neuron) influences the excitability of the second (the
postsynaptic neuron). At the synapse, the electric impulse is transformed
into a chemical form of transmission.

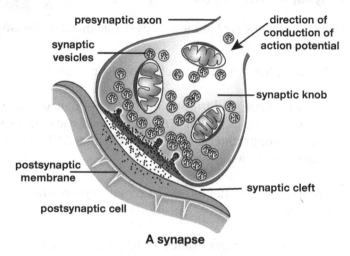

A synapse

Chemical transmission at the synapse involves the processes of
neurosecretion and chemoreception. The arrival of a nerve impulse at
the axon terminal stimulates the release of a specific chemical substance,
which has been synthesized in the cell body and stored in the tip of the
axon, into the narrow synaptic space between the adjacent neurons. This
process constitutes neurosecretion. The chemical secreted, known as
a neurotransmitter, can cause local depolarization of the membrane of
the postsynaptic region and thus transmit the excitation to the adjacent
neuron. Chemoreception is the process in which the neurotransmitter
becomes attached to specific molecular sites on the membrane of the
dendrite (postsynaptic region), producing a change in the properties of
the cell membrane so that a new impulse is established.

The chemical transmitter (for example, acetylcholine) passes from
the presynaptic axon to the postsynaptic dendrite by simple diffusion
across the narrow space, called the synaptic cleft, separating the two

neurons involved in the synapse. The synaptic clefts have been measured under the electron microscope to be about 200 angstrom in width. Diffusion is rapid enough to account for the speed of transmission observed at the synapse. After the neurotransmitter has exerted its effect on the postsynaptic membrane, it is promptly destroyed by an enzyme called cholinesterase. This destruction is of critical importance. If the acetylcholine were not destroyed, it would continue its stimulatory action indefinitely and all control would be lost.

8.3 Reflex Arc

The reflex arc is a simple neural pathway connecting receptors to an effector. A receptor detects a stimulus or environmental change. An effector is an organ of response (e.g., skeletal muscle). It produces a response called a reflex. This response does not involve the conscious involvement from higher centers in the brain. The reflex arc has five components that are activated in the following order:

Receptor - This specialized cell, or group of cells, detects a stimulus. During the knee-jerk (patellar) reflex, the patellar ligament (linking the patella to the tibia) is struck. This excites receptors in the tendon connecting the patella to the quadriceps muscle in the anterior thigh.

Sensory Neuron - This neuron sends impulses from the point of the stimulus to the CNS. For the knee-jerk reflex, and other spinal cord reflexes, sensory neurons enter the dorsal region of the cord.

Interneuron - This neuron in the CNS sends impulses from the sensory neuron to the motor neuron. The interneuron is separated from the other two neurons by synapses. For spinal cord reflexes, interneurons are located in the inner zone of gray matter.

Motor Neuron - This neuron sends impulses to the effector. For spinal cord reflexes, motor neurons exit from the ventral region of the spinal cord.

Effector - This organ carries out a response. During the knee-jerk response, the quadriceps muscle extends the lower leg.

Reflexes - These are automatic responses that depend on the activation of the components of the reflex arc. Some are coordinated by the spinal cord (e.g., knee jerk); others are coordinated by unconscious centers of the brain (e.g., dilation and constriction of the pupil of the eye).

Problem Solving Example:

 Describe and give an example of a reflex arc.

To understand what a reflex arc is, we must know something about reflexes. A reflex is an innate, stereotyped, automatic response to a given stimulus. A popular example of a reflex is the knee jerk. No matter how many times we rap on the tendon of a person's knee cap, his or her leg will invariably straighten out. This experiment demonstrates one of the chief characteristics of a reflex: fidelity of repetition.

Reflexes are important because responses to certain stimuli have to be made instantaneously. For example, when we step on something sharp or come into contact with something hot, we do not wait until the pain is experienced by the brain and then after deliberation decide what to do. Our responses are immediate and automatic. The part of the body involved is being withdrawn by reflex action before the sensation of pain is experienced.

A reflex arc is the neural pathway that conducts the nerve impulses for a given reflex. It consists of a sensory neuron with a receptor to detect the stimulus, connected by a synapse to a motor neuron, which is attached to a muscle or some other tissue that brings about the appropriate response. Thus, the simplest type of reflex arc is termed monosynaptic because there is only one synapse between the sensory and motor neurons. Most reflex arcs include one or more interneurons between the sensory and motor neurons (see figure on the next page).

An example of a monosynaptic reflex arc is the knee jerk. When the tendon of the knee cap is tapped, and thereby stretched, receptors

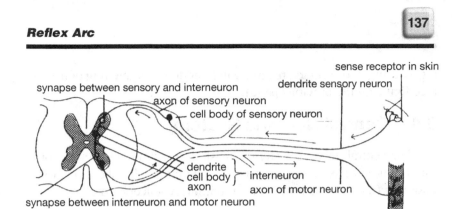

A reflex arc showing the pathway of an impulse, indicated by arrows

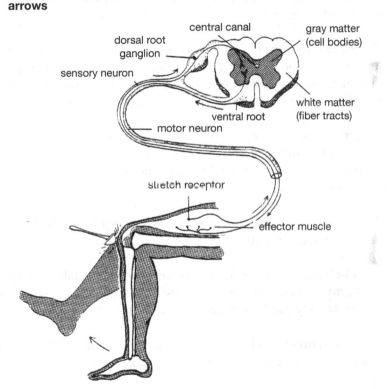

The knee-jerk reflex arc. The path of the impulse is indicated by arrows.

in the tendon are stimulated. An impulse travels along the sensory neuron to the spinal cord, where it synapses directly with a motor neuron. This latter neuron transmits an impulse to the effector muscle in the leg, causing it to contract, resulting in a sudden straightening of the leg (see figure on the previous page).

8.4 Central Nervous System

The central nervous system consists of the brain and spinal cord. The brain consists of several regions: hindbrain (rhombencephalon), midbrain (mesencephalon), and forebrain (prosencephalon).

8.4.1 Brain

The **hindbrain** consists of the medulla oblongata, pons, cerebellum, and fourth ventricle.

Medulla Oblongata - Continuous with the spinal cord, this is the most inferior portion of the brain. It contains vital centers: the respiratory, cardiac, and vasomotor (blood pressure) centers. It also coordinates many reflexes: vomiting, swallowing, coughing, and sneezing.

Tracts - This is a group of axons in the CNS that pass through the spinal cord and brain regions. The tracts, ascending and descending, are responsible for vertical relay throughout the CNS. Most of these tracts cross over at the level of the medulla.

Pons - This is a bulbous region that is superior to the medulla. It contains the tracts for vertical relay.

Cerebellum - The cerebellum is posterior to the medulla and pons. This butterfly-shaped structure is responsible for motor coordination. It also controls body equilibrium, posture, and muscle tone.

Fourth Ventricle - This is one of four such chambers throughout the brain. Each secretes and circulates cerebrospinal fluid (CSF).

The **midbrain** consists of the cerebral peduncles (two), the cerebral aqueduct, and the corpora quadrigemina.

Cerebral Peduncle - This is the stalk-like, anterior portion of the midbrain. Each peduncle contains tracts for vertical relay.

Cerebral Aqueduct - This is a passageway conducting the CSF from the third ventricle (in the forebrain) to the fourth ventricle.

Corpora Quadrigemina - This consists of four rounded structures called colliculi (singular, colliculus) that coordinate visual and auditory reflexes.

The **brainstem**, a vertical and unconscious portion of the brain, consists of the medulla, pons, and midbrain. The **forebrain** is mounted on it, much as the cap of a mushroom.

The **lower forebrain** (diencephalon) consists of the thalamus, hypothalamus, and third ventricle.

Thalamus - The thalamus is a mass of gray matter ranging through the roof of the third ventricle. It contains tracts for vertical relay. Serving as a screen or filter, it allows only some ascending signals to reach the higher forebrain.

Hypothalamus - This is a mass of gray matter forming the lateral walls and floor of the third ventricle. It contains centers for thirst, hunger, body temperature, and water balance. It signals the pituitary gland, which is attached to the floor of the third ventricle.

Third Ventricle - This chamber receives the CSF from the lateral ventricles in the higher forebrain (cerebrum).

The **cerebrum** is the **higher forebrain**. It consists of two halves or cerebral **hemispheres**. Its main features are:

Cortex - The cerebral cortex is the thin, wrinkled gray matter covering each hemisphere. The cortex has **convolutions** or gyruses, which are elevated areas of the cortex. A **sulcus** is a shallow groove between convolutions. A **fissure** is a deep groove. These markings greatly increase the surface area of the cortex.

Lobes - The cortex of each hemisphere is divided into four lobes. Each lobe has convolutions with mapped **sensory** and **motor** functions: **frontal** (motor: skeletal muscles, speech), **parietal** (sensory: skin and skeletal muscles), **temporal** (sensory: olfaction, taste, hearing), and **occipital** (sensory: vision). **Association areas** make up most of the cortex. They integrate functions between the sensory and motor areas, contributing abstract functions such as memory and reasoning.

White Matter - Each cerebral hemisphere contains a thick core of white matter containing myelinated axons that send signals. The **corpus callosum** is a bridge of white matter connecting the two hemispheres. Masses of gray matter (i.e., caudate nucleus) are located within the white matter. They control unconscious motor activity.

Ventricles - Each hemisphere contains a **lateral ventricle**. Each ventricle, or chamber, is inferior to the corpus callosum and secretes CSF through a foramen into the third ventricle.

Problem Solving Example:

 Label the principal parts of the human brain and list the function(s) carried out by each.

 The human brain is the enlarged, anterior end of the spinal cord. This enlargement is so great that the resemblance to the spinal

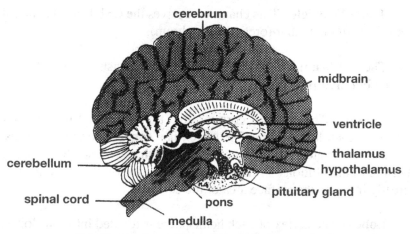

Interior portion of one side of the human brain

cord is obscured. The adult human brain has six major regions: the medulla, pons, and cerebellum, which constitute the hindbrain; the thalamus and cerebrum, both of which are in the forebrain; and the midbrain.

The most inferior part of the brain, connected immediately to the spinal cord, is the medulla. Here the central canal of the spinal cord (spinal lumen) enlarges to form a fluid-filled cavity called the fourth ventricle. The medulla has numerous nerve tracts (bundles of nerves) that bring impulses to and from the brain. The medulla also contains a number of clusters of nerve cell bodies, known as nerve centers. These reflex centers control respiration, heart rate, the dilation and constriction of blood vessels, swallowing, and vomiting.

Above the medulla is the cerebellum, which is made up of a central part and two hemispheres that extend sideways. The size of the cerebellum in different animals is roughly correlated with the amount of their muscular activity. The cerebellum regulates and coordinates muscle contraction. Removal or injury of the cerebellum is accompanied not by paralysis of the muscles but by impairment of muscle coordination.

The pons is an area of the hindbrain containing a large number of nerve fibers, which pass through it and make connections between the two hemispheres of the cerebellum, thus coordinating muscle movements on the two sides of the body. The pons also contains the nerve centers that aid in the regulation of breathing.

In front of the cerebellum and pons lies the thickwalled midbrain. The midbrain is an important integrating region and contains the centers for certain visual and auditory reflexes. A cluster of nerve cells regulating muscle tone and posture is also present in the midbrain. A small canal runs through the midbrain and connects the fourth ventricle behind it to the third ventricle in front of it.

The midbrain, pons, and medulla are collectively called the brainstem. Ten of the twelve cranial nerves originate in the brainstem.

The thalamus of the forebrain serves as a relay center for sensory impulses. Fibers from the spinal cord and parts of the brain synapse here with other neurons going to the various sensory areas of the cerebrum. The thalamus seems to regulate and coordinate the external signs of emotions. By stimulating the thalamus with an electrode, a sham rage can be elicited in a cat—the hair stands on end, the claws protrude, and the back becomes humped. However, as soon as the stimulation ceases, the rage responses disappear.

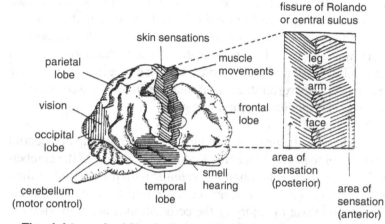

The right cerebral hemisphere of the human brain, seen from the side. The striped areas are regions of special function; the light areas are "association" areas. Inset: Enlarged view of the sensory and motor areas adjacent to the fissure of Rolando, showing the location of the nerve cells supplying the various parts of the body.

The hypothalamus, located under the thalamus, is a collection of nuclei (a cluster of nerve cell bodies located within the central nervous system) concerned with many important homeostatic regulations. Electrical stimulation of certain cells in the hypothalamus produces sensations of hunger, thirst, pain, pleasure, or sexual drive. The hypothalamus is also important for its influence on the pituitary gland, which is functionally under its control. Cells of the hypothalamus synthesize chemical factors that modulate the release of hormones produced and stored in the anterior pituitary. The hypothalamus has neural connections with the posterior pituitary. The hypothalamus and thalamus are collectively called the diencephalon.

The cerebrum, consisting of two hemispheres, is the largest and most anterior part of the human brain. In human beings, the cerebral hemispheres grow back over the rest of the brain, hiding it from view. Each hemisphere contains one cavity (one contains the first and the other the second ventricle, collectively known as the lateral ventricles), which is connected to the third ventricle. The outer portion of the cerebral hemisphere, the cortex, is made up of gray matter that comprises the nerve cell bodies. The gray matter folds greatly, producing many convolutions of the cerebral surface. These convolutions increase the surface area of the gray matter. The inner part of the brain is the white matter that is composed of masses of nerve fibers.

Each cerebral hemisphere is divided into four lobes. The occipital or posterior lobe receives visual information. The temporal lobe, located on the side of the cerebrum just above the ears, receives auditory information. The frontal and parietal lobes are demarcated by the fissure of Rolando. Just in front of this fissure in the frontal lobe is the primary motor area, while the primary sensory area lies behind it in the parietal lobe.

When all the areas of known functions are plotted, they cover only a small part of the total area of the human cortex. The rest, known as association areas, are regions responsible for the higher intellectual faculties of memory, reasoning, learning, and imagination, all of which help to make up one's personality. In some unknown way, the association regions integrate into a meaningful unit, with all the diverse impulses constantly reaching the brain, so that the proper response is made.

8.4.2 Spinal Cord

The spinal cord consists of two halves, divided by an anterior fissure and posterior sulcus. It contains regions of white matter and gray matter. Each performs one function.

White Matter - The white matter is external. On each side of the cord, these myelinated axons are organized into **columns: anterior, lateral**, and **posterior**. The columns contain tracts for vertical relay. For example, the spinothalamic is an ascending tract. The corticospinal is a descending tract.

Gray Matter - The gray matter is internal, appearing much as a butterfly in flight. On each side it is organized into **horns: anterior**, **lateral**, and **posterior**. The horns contain interneurons that complete reflex arcs coordinated by the cord.

The brain and spinal cord are covered by several layers of **meninges** (singular, **meninx**): the **dura mater** (external layer), **arachnoid mater** (middle layer), and **pia mater** (internal layer adhering to nerve tissue).

Problem Solving Example:

 Describe the structures found in a cross section of the spinal cord.

 The spinal cord extends from the base of the brain and is tubular in shape. Along with the brain, the spinal cord makes up the central nervous system of all vertebrates. It has two very important functions: to transmit impulses to and from the brain and to act as a reflex center.

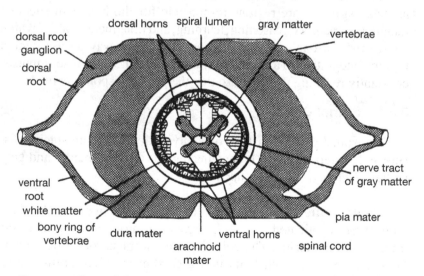

Cross section of the mammalian spinal cord surrounded by the bony vertebrae

The spinal cord is protected by the vertebral column. The vertebral column is composed of segments of bone, called the vertebrae, connected to each other by cartilage. The cartilage gives it flexibility, while the bone gives it strength. It is possible to anatomically divide the spinal cord into five different regions using the vertebrae as a guide. These are the (1) cervical region, (2) thoracic region, (3) lumbar region, (4) sacral region, and (5) coccygeal region. The regions of the spinal cord send out nerves that innervate different parts of the body.

The spinal cord is surrounded by three membranes: the dura mater, arachnoid mater, and pia mater. It is a hollow, tubular structure. The hollow portion, called the spinal lumen, runs through the entire length of the spinal cord and is filled with spinal fluid. A cross section shows two regions: an inner mass of gray matter composed of nerve cell bodies and an outer mass of white matter made up of bundles of axons and dendrites. The coloration of the white matter region is due to the presence of white myelinated fibers. The nerve cells of the gray matter lack myelin, which is white, and hence the natural gray color of nerve cells is seen. Four protuberances of the gray matter are noted. The two anterior processes are called the ventral horns, and the two posterior ones are called the dorsal horns. The axons and dendrites of the white matter carry impulses between lower levels and higher levels of the spinal cord, or between various levels of the spinal cord and the brain.

The spinal cord receives sensory fibers from peripheral receptors at the dorsal root. The cell bodies from which the sensory fibers arise are located in a cluster, called the dorsal root ganglion, in the dorsal root. These sensory fibers pass into the dorsal horns of the gray matter, where they synapse with interneurons in the dorsal horns and/or motor neurons in the ventral horns. Axons from the motor neurons leave the spinal cord at the ventral root and soon join the sensory fibers—together they constitute the spinal nerve. Spinal nerves arise from the spinal cord branch to supply various parts of the body except the head, part of the neck, the thorax, abdomen, and the upper and lower extremities.

8.5   Peripheral Nervous System

Among the 12 pairs of cranial nerves, some contain only motor neurons. Some are purely sensory. Others are mixed, containing sensory and motor neurons.

8.5.1   Cranial Nerves and Spinal Nerves

The cranial nerve pairs are numbered one through twelve in a posterior direction as they connect to the brain. Their main functions are:

I.   **Olfactory** - sense of smell, sensory nerve

II.   **Optic** - sense of vision, sensory nerve

III.   **Oculomotor** - moves the eye, motor nerve

IV.   **Trochlear** - moves the eye, motor nerve

V.   **Trigeminal** - sensory for teeth, eyes, tongue; motor for muscles of mastication (chewing)

VI.   **Abducens** - moves the eye, motor nerve

VII.   **Facial** - sensory for taste; motor for facial muscles and salivary glands

VIII.   **Vestibulocochlear** - balance and hearing, sensory nerve

IX.   **Glossopharyngeal** - sensory and motor for tongue

X.   **Vagus** - sensory and motor for internal organs

XI.   **Spinal Accessory** - motor for muscles of neck and shoulder

XII.   **Hypoglossal** - motor for the tongue

Spinal Nerves - All 31 pairs of spinal nerves are mixed. They are organized into the following groups:

Cervical - 8 pairs

Thoracic - 12 pairs

Lumbar - 5 pairs

Sacral - 5 pairs

Coccygeal - 1 pair

Branches of many of the spinal nerves form complex networks called **plexuses**. For example, the cervical plexus (pairs C1 through C4) controls the skin and muscles of the neck plus the diaphragm. The brachial plexus (C5 through T1) controls the skin and muscles of the arms.

Spinal nerve–spinal cord functions on one side of the body are controlled by the cerebral cortex on the opposite side. For example, the right hemisphere controls the left arm. This is because the tracts for vertical relay through the CNS cross over at the medulla.

Problem Solving Examples:

Q There are 12 pairs of cranial nerves in humans. Give the type(s) of fibers found in each and briefly discuss the function(s) of each of them.

A Cranial nerves leave the brain from different regions and serve different functions. They connect the brain to various effector organs, primarily the sense organs, muscles, and glands of the head. Some cranial nerves contain only motor fibers, some contain only sensory fibers, and some contain both types of fibers. In addition, some are composed of parasympathetic fibers (which are exclusively motor), the action of which is involuntary.

There are 12 pairs of cranial nerves in humans. The olfactory nerve (cranial nerve I) is composed entirely of afferent fibers carrying impulses for the sense of smell from the olfactory epithelium to the base of the brain. The optic nerve (II) is also entirely sensory and contains afferent fibers running from the retina to the visual center of the brain. The oculomotor (III) and trochlear (IV) nerves both have afferent and efferent branches that connect the midbrain to the muscles of the eye.

Together they are responsible for proprioception of the eye muscles, movement of the eyeball, accommodation of the eye, and constriction of the pupil. The trigeminal nerve (V) contains both afferent and efferent fibers running between the pons and the face and jaws. It functions mainly in stimulating movement of the muscles of the jaws involved in chewing. The fibers of the abducens nerve (VI) run between the pons and muscles of the eye. This nerve conveys the sense of position of the eyeball to the brain, and aids the III and IV nerves in effecting movement of the eyeball.

The facial nerve (VII) has both afferent and efferent fibers that innervate muscles of the face, mouth, forehead, and scalp. It also functions in the transmission of impulses for the sense of taste from the anterior part of the tongue to the brain. The fibers of the auditory nerve or vestibulocochlear nerve (VIII), exclusively afferent, run from the inner ear to the junction of the pons and medulla. These fibers convey the senses of hearing and equilibrium (movement, balance, and rotation) to the appropriate centers in the brain. Connecting the medulla to the epithelium and muscles of the pharynx, and to the salivary gland and tongue, are the fibers of the glossopharyngeal nerve (IX). This nerve is responsible for the sense of taste from the posterior part of the tongue and from the lining of the larynx. It is also responsible for the reflexive act of swallowing.

The tenth cranial nerve, the vagus (X), has both sensory and motor branches, but the motor fibers are parasympathetic autonomic fibers and thus their action is involuntary. Its sensory fibers originate in many of the internal organs—lungs, stomach, aorta, larynx, to name a few— and its motor (parasympathetic) fibers run to the heart, stomach, small intestine, larynx, and esophagus. Besides the vagus, the III, VII, and IX nerves also contain parasympathetic fibers, but in smaller amounts. The efferent and afferent branches of the spinal accessory nerve (XI) connect the medulla to the pharynx and larynx and muscles of the shoulder, which they innervate. Afferent fibers of the last cranial nerve, the hypoglossal, convey the sense of proprioception from the tongue to the medulla, and the efferent fibers stimulate movement of the tongue.

The cranial nerves are numbered anteriorly to posteriorly. I and II originate in the olfactory epithelium and retina, respectively. III and IV originate in the midbrain; V through VIII (vestibular branch) originate in the pons; and VIII (cochlear branch) through XII originate in the medulla.

 What are spinal nerves, and what are their functions?

Spinal nerves belong to the peripheral nervous system (PNS). They arise as pairs at regular intervals from the spinal cord, branch, and run to various parts of the body to innervate them. In human beings, there are 31 symmetrical pairs of spinal nerves. The size of each spinal nerve is related to the size of the body area it innervates.

All the spinal nerves are mixed nerves, in the sense that all have both motor and sensory components in roughly equal amounts. They contain fibers of the somatic nervous system, which are both afferent (conducting impulses towards the nervous system) and efferent (conducting impulses to effector organs). They also contain fibers of the autonomic nervous system, which are uniquely efferent and are separable into parasympathetic and sympathetic nervous systems. Because of this nature, the spinal nerves function to convey messages from the external environment to the central nervous system and from the central nervous system to various effectors of the body. In other words, the spinal nerves, as part of the peripheral nervous system, serve as a link between the central nervous system and the effector organs.

Somatic fibers of the spinal nerves innervate skeletal muscles of the body and are under voluntary regulation. We can bend our arm or leg at will. The autonomic nerves innervate the smooth and cardiac muscles and glands of the body and cannot be voluntarily controlled. We cannot speed up our stomach contractions or heartbeat at will. The autonomic nerve fibers leave the spinal cord and run for a certain distance with the somatic fibers in the spinal nerves. Then the two types of fibers diverge and run to their respective body areas, which they innervate.

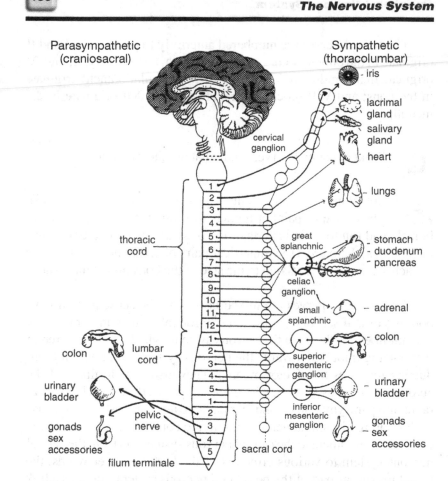

The spinal nerves and their autonomic fibers. The somatic fibers leave the spinal cord together with the autonomic fibers and then separate.

8.5.2 Autonomic Nervous System

The autonomic nervous system (ANS) controls motor functions of the internal organs (smooth, cardiac muscle) and glands. It consists of two branches:

Sympathetic - This branch includes fibers of thoracic and lumbar nerves. The nerves have preganglionic and postganglionic neurons. The postganglionic neurons discharge a neurotransmitter called **norepinephrine** at the synapses meeting internal organs.

Parasympathetic - This branch includes fibers of cranial and sacral nerves. The nerves also have preganglionic and postganglionic neurons, but the postganglionic cells discharge **acetylcholine** as the terminal transmitter.

Both branches control the activity of an internal organ at any time. However, the sympathetic branch dominates during the "**fight-or-flight**" response of the body. This is appropriate during stressful or hyperactive states of the body (e.g., exercise). Therefore, the sympathetic effect increases the following: rate of heartbeat, rate and depth of breathing, bloodflow to most skeletal muscles, and concentration of glucose in the blood. However, it also decreases certain processes: bloodflow to digestive organs and digestion.

The parasympathetic effect is the opposite of the sympathetic effect on an internal organ (e.g., decreases rate of heartbeat, increases digestion). This branch normally restores a normal, more relaxed state to body processes.

Problem Solving Example:

Q What is meant by the autonomic nervous system? What are its subdivisions and to which of the large divisions of the entire nervous system does it belong?

A Nerves from the central nervous system (CNS) that innervate the cardiac muscles, smooth muscles, and secretory glands form the autonomic nervous system. Structural and physiological differences within the autonomic nervous system are the basis for its further subdivision into sympathetic and parasympathetic systems. Nerves of these two divisions leave the CNS at different regions. The sympathetic nerves emerge from the thoracic and lumbar regions of the spinal cord, and the parasympathetic nerves arise from the brainstem and sacral portions of the spinal cord. Thus, the sympathetic system is known as the thoracolumbar outflow (originating in T_1–T_{12} and L_1–L_2), while the parasympathetic system is referred to as the craniosacral outflow (originating in cranial nerves III, VII, IX, and sacral nerves 2 through 4).

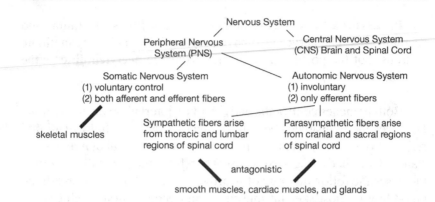

Summary of the divisions and subdivisions of the mammalian nervous system

The autonomic nervous system contains only motor nerves and is distinguished from the rest of the nervous system by several characteristics. There is no voluntary control by the cerebrum over these nerves. We cannot control the action of the muscles of the stomach or intestines, but can, in some cases, slow our heartbeat. Another important characteristic of the autonomic nervous system is that most internal organs receive a double set of fibers, one set belonging to the sympathetic system and the other to the parasympathetic system. Impulses from the sympathetic and parasympathetic nerves always have antagonistic effects on the organs innervated. Thus, if one functions to increase a certain activity, the other functions to decrease it. However, many tissues/cells do not receive parasympathetic innervation (e.g., fat cells, most arterioles, spleen).

The autonomic nervous system is part of a larger unit called the peripheral nervous system. The peripheral nervous system contains two types of nerve fibers: the afferent fibers that convey information from receptors in the periphery to the CNS, and the efferent fibers that carry information from the CNS to the effectors. Effectors are tissues or organs that bring about appropriate responses to certain stimuli, both internal (i.e., from the brain) and external (i.e., from the environment). Some examples of effectors are the skeletal muscles, cardiac and smooth muscles, and secretory glands. The peripheral nervous system can be divided functionally into two parts. That part that innervates the skeletal muscles is known as the somatic nervous system, and that which innervates smooth muscle, cardiac muscle, and glands is the autonomic nervous system.

Quiz: The Nervous System

1. Which of the following is not involved in the process of synaptic transmission?

    (A) The release of a neurotransmitter from synaptic vesicles at the presynaptic neuron

    (B) The destruction of the postsynaptic membrane after the neurotransmitter has come into contact with it

    (C) Diffusion of the neurotransmitter across the synaptic cleft

    (D) Destruction of the neurotransmitter after transmission of the impulse has taken place

    (E) None of the above.

2. The most common neurotransmitter of vertebrate neuromuscular synapses is

    (A) epinephrine.

    (B) acetylcholine.

    (C) norepinephrine.

    (D) serotonin.

    (E) dopamine.

3. Which of the following is present in the synaptic vesicles?

    (A) Action potential

    (B) Neurotransmitters

    (C) Na^+

    (D) Synaptic inhibitors

    (E) K^+

4. The part of the brain that regulates and coordinates muscle movement is the

    (A) cerebellum.

    (B) pons.

    (C) ventricle.

    (D) medulla.

    (E) thalamus.

5. Which of the following are not innervated by the autonomic nervous system?

    (A) Leg muscles

    (B) Pupillary muscles

    (C) Adrenal glands

    (D) Pituitary glands

    (E) Heart muscles

6. Which of the following best describes the major function(s) of the spinal cord?

    (A) Acts as a messenger to the brain

    (B) Filters sensory impulses

    (C) Directs simple actions independent of brain

    (D) Both (A) and (B).

    (E) Both (A) and (C).

7. A nervous impulse starting at the dendrite will next pass through the

    (A) cell body.

    (B) axon.

(C) nodes of Ranvier.

    (D) synaptic button.

    (E) None of the above.

8.   If one were to cut the parasympathetic nerve (vagus) that innervates the heart, one would expect to see

    (A) an increase in heart rate due to increased sympathetic activity.

    (B) an increase in heart rate due to decreased parasympathetic activity.

    (C) a decrease in heart rate due to decreased parasympathetic activity.

    (D) a dead heart, as a heart requires innervation for function.

    (E) a decrease in heart rate, since that is the effect of parasympathetic stimulation.

9.   Select the function not performed by the temporal lobe of the brain.

    (A) Gestation

    (B) Hearing

    (C) Smell

    (D) Taste

    (E) Vision

10. Concerning the development of the vertebrate brain,

    (A) the prosencephalon consists of the pons and cerebellum.

    (B) the mesencephalon develops into the myelencephalon and metencephalon.

(C)   the rhombencephalon consists of the pons, medulla oblongata, and cerebellum.

   (D)   the telencephalon develops into the prosencephalon and diencephalon.

   (E)   the cerebellum is part of the diencephalon.

ANSWER KEY

1.	(B)	6.	(E)
2.	(B)	7.	(A)
3.	(B)	8.	(B)
4.	(A)	9.	(E)
5.	(A)	10.	(C)

CHAPTER 9

The Sense Organs

9.1 Receptors

Receptors are specialized cells that can detect environmental changes called stimuli. Sense organs contain receptors. The skin, for example, is a sense organ that contains receptors that detect a wide variety of stimuli for touch, pressure, heat, cold, and pain.

Chemoreceptors detect chemical stimuli. These receptors are responsible for the senses of taste and olfaction. Each of the receptors for the four basic tastes (salty, sour, bitter, and sweet) are concentrated over different regions on the surface of the tongue. Different receptors in the epithelium of the upper nasal mucosa are responsible for the different senses of olfaction.

Proprioceptors are located in the joints of the body with tendons and ligaments. They are sensitive to stretching and pressure. They contribute to a person's knowledge of the position of body parts. The knee-jerk reflex begins with the stimulation of proprioceptors.

The retina of the eye contains **photoreceptors** (rods and cones) that are sensitive to light. The **mechanoreceptors** (sensory hair cells) of the inner ear are responsible for balance and hearing.

The development of any sense requires the activation of three components: (1) the stimulation of receptors, (2) impulse transmission by associated sensory neurons to the spinal cord and/or brain, and (3) interpretation of the sensory input by a mapped sensory area of the cerebral cortex.

The sense of vision develops by the activation of all three components. Retinal cells are stimulated. This activates sensory neurons of the optic nerve. Impulses along these neurons enter the brain and arrive at a mapped area on the cortex of the occipital lobe for interpretation.

9.2   Eye

The eye is a sensory organ with receptors located in its innermost layer, the retina. Several associated or accessory structures work with the eye for vision.

9.2.1   Associated Structures

Orbit - This is the eye socket. Seven different skull bones (e.g., frontal, maxilla, zygomatic) of the orbit are joined by sutures to house and protect most of the eye.

Extrinsic Muscles - Six skeletal muscles are attached to the eye. Four of the muscles have fibers ranging straight through the orbit (rectus = straight): **lateral rectus, medial rectus, superior rectus,** and **inferior rectus**. Two of the muscles have fibers ranging obliquely: **superior oblique** and **inferior oblique**. When each muscle contracts, it moves the eye in a specific direction. For example, the eye moves in a lateral direction when the lateral rectus contracts.

These muscles are controlled by motor neurons of cranial nerves III, IV, and VI (oculomotor, trochlear, and abducens).

Palpebra - The palpebra is the eyelid. A skeletal muscle inside the eyelid, the **levator palpebra**, contracts to raise the eyelid and open the eye. The **orbicularis oculi**, a series of circular muscle fibers around the front margin of the orbit, contract to oppose this action and close the eye.

The palpebra has an outer layer of skin. The inner surface is lined by the **conjunctiva**, a mucous membrane that doubles back over the exposed surface of the eye (cornea and part of the sclera). Eyelashes are attached to the edge of the palpebra.

Lacrimal Apparatus - The lacrimal apparatus is a series of structures that form, secrete, and drain the lacrimal fluid (tear fluid). The **lacrimal gland**, embedded in the frontal bone above the eye, secretes the fluid through a group of **lacrimal ducts**. The fluid washes over the exposed surface of the eye, lubricating and moistening this surface. Two small ducts drain the fluid in the medial corner, passing it to the **nasolacrimal duct**. From this duct, the fluid enters the **lacrimal sac**.

9.2.2 Structure of the Eye

Most of the makeup of the eye consists of several layers. The balance of the anatomy consists of three internal, transparent structures.

Sclera - Also known as the scleroid coat, this is the outer white covering of the eye. It provides protection much as the leathery cover protects a baseball.

Cornea - The sclera is modified anteriorly into a clear, centrally located layer called the cornea. This convex layer is the first structure to intercept light rays. Its convexity allows it to refract (bend) these rays, concentrating them as they are collected to fall on the retina inside.

Choroid Coat - This dark, middle layer is highly vascular. The blood vessels deliver nutrients and oxygen to the tissues of the eye. The choroid coat is modified into three structures anteriorly.

Ciliary Body/Suspensory Ligaments - The choroid coat thickens anteriorly into a ring of smooth muscle, the ciliary body. Suspensory ligaments continue from it, attaching to the lens. The lens is a convex structure that is also elastic. Its convexity is determined by the degree of tension placed on it by the ciliary body and attached ligaments. The convexity will change for viewing objects at varying distances.

Iris - The iris is the third anterior modification of the middle layer. Anterior to the ciliary body, the iris is a ring consisting of two layers of smooth muscle, circular and radial, that surround an opening called the **pupil**. If a viewed area becomes brighter, contraction of the circular fibers constrict the pupil. If the area becomes darker, contraction of the radial fibers dilates the pupil. Therefore, the size of the pupil controls the amount of light passing through the eye.

Retina - The retina is the inner lining, covering about the posterior three-quarters of the eye. It does not have any anterior modifications. The retina contains two kinds of photoreceptors, **rods** and **cones**.

The cones are active in bright light and are responsible for color discrimination and the formation of sharp images. Color vision depends on the interaction of cones with three kinds of pigments—red, blue, and green. The concentration of cones is greatest in the **fovea centralis** (focal point) on the retina.

Rods contain rhodopsin, a pigment that becomes active during dim-light conditions. Their concentration increases with increasing distance from the focal point, just the opposite of the pattern for the cones. The rods are responsible for black and white vision.

The **optic disc** (blind spot) is a retinal region somewhat off center from the location of the focal point. Photoreceptors are absent here, as there is an opening for the passage of neurons of the **optic nerve**.

Lens - The lens is one of several transparent structures. It is a biconvex, elastic structure connected to the suspensory ligaments. Its convexity allows it to refract light rays.

Aqueous Humor - This is a fluid filling the anterior chamber of the eye. It is constantly being formed from capillaries in the ciliary body. It is drained by a circular canal (canal of Schlemm) where the sclera meets the cornea.

Vitreous Body (Humor) - This is a gelatin-like substance filling the larger posterior chamber. It maintains the shape of the eyeball. Its amount remains stable. Unlike the aqueous humor, it is not constantly drained and reformed.

9.2.3 Physiology of Vision

Light passes through the following sequence of structures before falling on the retina: **cornea**, **aqueous humor**, **lens**, **vitreous body**, **retina**. Each of these structures has the ability to refract light rays. Because of their convex shape, the cornea and lens bend the rays by causing their convergence. This is necessary, as light rays tend to scatter and diverge from any point on a viewed object. Through convergence the light rays are collected and concentrated.

The majority of rays from any point of an object fall on or near the fovea centralis of the retina. The maximum concentration of cones is found here for maximum sensory ability and sharp image formation.

The convexity of the lens changes for viewing objects at varying distances. The pattern of response is:

closer object, more convexity, more convergence of rays
more distant object, less convexity, less convergence of rays

Light rays diverge more from closer objects; therefore, the convexity and refractive power of the lens must increase. For more distant objects, light rays do not diverge as much. In this case, the refractive power of the lens does not need to be as great, and it flattens out somewhat, becoming less convex. The change in the shape of the lens for viewing objects of varying distances is called **accommodation**.

Problem Solving Examples:

 Draw a diagram of the human eye, labeling all parts. Briefly describe the function of each part.

 The human eye consists of three layers or tunics. The fibrous tunic is the outermost layer of the eye: it consists of the sclera

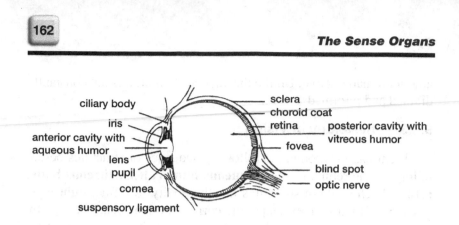

ciliary body — sclera — choroid coat
iris — retina — posterior cavity with vitreous humor
anterior cavity with aqueous humor — fovea
lens
pupil — blind spot
cornea — optic nerve
suspensory ligament

Cross section of the human eye

posteriorly and the cornea anteriorly. The sclera is a protective coat and is the "white of the eye." The cornea is the transparent covering that functions in the refraction (bending) of light.

The middle coat is the vascular layer. Posteriorly, it consists of the choroid coat. This pigmented layer absorbs excess light and nourishes the retina through its rich vasculature. The choroid continues anteriorly as the ciliary body. The ciliary body consists of the ciliary muscle, a smooth muscle that functions in the accommodation reflex, and the ciliary process that secretes aqueous humor (fluid) into the anterior part of the eye. Finally, the ciliary body continues anteriorly as the iris. The iris is the colored part of the eye and also contains smooth muscle that functions in controlling the size of the pupil—the small opening through which light passes.

The innermost layer is the nervous tunic. It consists solely of the retina in the back of the eye. The retina consists of photoreceptor cells called rods and cones. In the center of the retina is a small depressed area called the fovea centralis, the region of keenest vision. Medial to this is the optic disc. The optic nerve exits the back of the eye at this point. Because there are no photoreceptors at the disc, there is a blind spot in the peripheral field of vision. There is no anterior continuation of the retina.

There are two fluid-filled cavities inside the eye. The anterior cavity contains an aqueous humor (a watery fluid) and is located between the cornea and the lens. The posterior cavity is filled with vitreous humor (a gel-like fluid) and is located between the lens and the retina. The transparent lens that separates these two cavities is responsible for focusing incoming light rays on the retina.

 Discuss the mechanism by which the photoreceptors are stimulated by light. How are rods and cones distributed in the retina?

Photoreceptors are sensory cells that are sensitive to light. In the human retina, they are called rods and cones according to their shapes. Both types of cells contain light-sensitive molecules called visual pigments whose primary function is to absorb light. The rods contain rhodopsin (visual purple), which is composed of a chromophore (a variant of vitamin A) and a protein (opsin). The cones contain iodopsin, which is made up of the same chromophore as in rhodopsin but with a different protein.

Light from the outside enters the eye and stimulates the rods or cones, thus triggering the emission of nerve impulses by the receptor cells. Light does not directly provide the necessary energy to set off the impulse. The energy comes from the chemical bonds in the rhodopsin or iodopsin molecule. In this respect, the phenomenon of vision is basically different from the phenomenon of photosynthesis, in which light supplies the energy to drive the series of chemical reactions.

When light strikes the visual pigments, it acts upon the chromophore, which then splits away from the opsin. This splitting occurs because light changes the molecular configuration of the chromophore in such a way that it no longer can bind to the opsin. Simultaneously, impulses are triggered, and these travel to the brain (via the optic nerve), where they are interpreted.

Rhodopsin is sensitive to a very small amount of light. Rod cells, which contain this kind of visual pigment, are used to detect objects in poor illumination, such as in night vision. They are not responsible for color vision, but are important in the perception of shades of gray and brightness. Their acuity — the ability to distinguish one point in space from another nearby point — is very poor. Rods are most numerous in the peripheral retina, that is, that part closest to the lens, and are absent from the very center of the retina (the fovea). On the other hand, cones operate only at high levels of illumination and are used for day vision. The primary function of the cones is to perceive colors. Their visual acuity is very high, and because they are concentrated in the center of the retina, it is that part that we use for fine, detailed vision.

9.3   Ear

The ear is responsible for hearing and two types of body equilibrium (balance). It consists of three regions: the external ear, middle ear, and inner ear.

9.3.1   Structure

External Ear - The external ear consists of the **pinna (auricle)** and **external auditory meatus** (auditory canal). The pinna is the outer ear flap, consisting of elastic cartilage covered with skin. The meatus is a tube passing from the pinna into the temporal bone. Vibrating air waves (sound waves) pass through here as they travel toward the middle ear.

Middle Ear - The middle ear begins at the **tympanic membrane** (eardrum). The **malleus** (hammer) is a middle ear bone attached to this membrane. If the tympanum vibrates from the arrival and impact of air waves, the malleus transmits the vibrations to the **incus** (anvil) and **stapes** (stirrups). The stapes is attached to the **oval window** of the inner ear. The vibration of the stapes transmits a signal to this membrane.

The **eustachian tube** is a passageway extending from the middle ear to the nasopharynx, which is part of the throat. Air moved through this tube, by yawning or swallowing, can restore a pressure balance on the tympanum. The eustachian tube, however, is not involved in the transmission of vibrations for hearing.

Inner Ear - The inner ear is a complex series of channels. The **cochlea** is the part containing the receptors for hearing. It contains three channels: the **vestibular canal** (scala vestibuli), **tympanic canal** (scala tympani), and **cochlear duct** (canal). The vestibular and tympanic canals are connected at their ends.

As vibrations arrive at the oval window from the middle ear, they continue through **perilymph**, a fluid in the vestibular canal and tympanic canal. From the tympanic canal, vibrations are sent to the **round window**. This membrane is the last structure to receive vibrations, serving as a shock absorber.

As vibrations pass through the perilymph, they disturb fluid, called **endolymph,** in the nearby cochlear duct. The cochlear duct contains the receptors, sensory hair cells, for hearing.

Two other structures of the inner ear, the **vestibule** and **semicircular** (half circle) **canals**, are involved with body equilibrium. The vestibule contains two small chambers, the **utricle** and **saccule**, that contain the receptors for static equilibrium. This involves balance when the body is relatively motionless. The three semicircular canals contain the receptors for dynamic equilibrium, maintaining balance when a person is moving.

9.3.2 Physiology of Hearing and Equilibrium

The original stimuli for hearing are vibrating sound waves. They pass through the structures of the ear in the following order: **auricle, external auditory meatus, tympanum, malleus, incus, stapes, oval window, vestibular canal, tympanic canal, round window**. As each of these structures vibrates, it normally maintains the frequency (pitch) of the original sound waves in the air. The three bones of the middle ear amplify the vibrations, causing them to sound louder.

As the perilymph in the vestibular and tympanic canals transmits the vibrations, it disturbs the endolymph and sensory hair cells in the cochlear duct. The hair cells are receptors, mounted on a **basilar membrane** and suspended in the endolymph. As the cells rub against the nearby **tectorial membrane**, a stimulus is produced. The sensory hair cells, plus the basilar and tectorial membranes, compose the **organ of Corti**.

Action potentials from the sensory neurons of the **cochlear nerve** of cranial nerve VIII (vestibulocochlear) are transmitted to the temporal lobe of the cerebral cortex, where they are interpreted as sound.

For static equilibrium, the saccule and utricle are lined with sensory hair cells suspended in a gelatin-like matrix. Small deposits of calcium carbonate, called otoliths, contact different groups of hair cells depending on the position of the body. These stimuli are conducted to the brain for interpretation.

For dynamic equilibrium, sensory hair cells line the ampullae (expanded regions) where the semicircular canals meet the vestibule. They contact a gelatin-like matrix inside. There are three canals on each side of the body. The canals are at right angles to each other. Based on the changing direction and position of the body when moving, different groups of hair cells are affected in different combinations. This information is conducted to the brain.

Sensory neurons of the **vestibular nerve** transmit signals from the vestibule and semicircular canals. Combined with the cochlear nerve fibers for hearing, they form the vestibulocochlear nerve. The cerebellum is one brain region receiving an input for body balance.

Problem Solving Example:

 With the aid of a diagram, describe the structures found in the human ear.

 Three parts of the human ear can be distinguished: the outer ear, the middle ear, and the inner ear. The outer ear consists of the skin-covered cartilaginous flap, or pinna, and a channel known as the

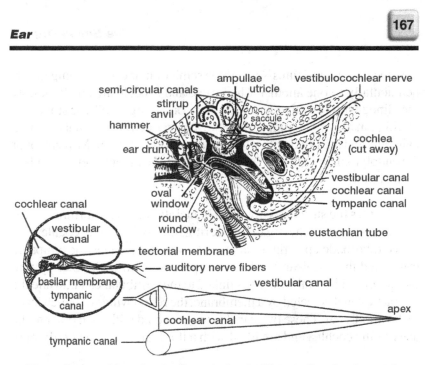

The coiled cochlea shown dissected out of the skull and cut open to reveal the vestibular canals (upper right). A diagram of the cochlea as though it were uncoiled and drawn out in a straight line (lower right). A cross section through the cochlea to show the organ of Corti resting on the basilar membrane and covered by the tectorial membrane (lower left).

external auditory meatus. At the inner end of this canal is a membrane called the tympanic membrane (eardrum).

On the other side of the tympanic membrane is a small chamber, the middle ear, which contains three tiny bones. These three bones are the malleus (hammer), incus (anvil), and stapes (stirrup), and are arranged in sequence across the middle ear from the tympanic membrane to another membrane, the oval window, which separates the middle ear from the inner ear. The middle ear is connected to the pharynx via the eustachian tube, which serves to equalize the air pressure between the outer and middle ear.

The inner ear consists of a complicated labyrinth of interconnected fluid-filled chambers and canals. One group of chambers and canals is involved with the sense of equilibrium. There are two small chambers—

the sacculus and utriculus—and three semicircular canals arranged per-
pendicularly to one another. The utricle and saccule are small, hollow
sacs lined with sensitive hair cells and containing small ear stones, or
otoliths, made of calcium carbonate. The semicircular canals contain
hair cells and are filled with a fluid known as endolymph. Movement of
the endolymph over the hair cells stimulates the latter to send impulses
to the brain.

Besides the structures involved in maintaining equilibrium, the inner ear also houses the organ for hearing, the cochlea. The cochlea is a
coiled tube made up of three canals—the vestibular canal, the tympanic
canal, and the cochlear canal, each separated from each other by thin
membranes. The oval window is linked to the vestibular canal, while the
tympanic canal is sealed by a membrane, the round window, which leads
to the middle ear. These two canals are connected with each other at the
apex of the cochlea and are filled with a fluid known as the perilymph.

The cochlear canal, filled with endolymph, contains the actual organ
of hearing, the organ of Corti. The organ of Corti consists of a layer of
epithelium, the basilar membrane, on which lie five rows of specialized
receptor cells extending the entire length of the coiled cochlea. Each
receptor cell is equipped with hair-like projections extending into the
cochlear canal. Overhanging the hair cells is a gelatinous structure, the
tectorial membrane, into which the hairs project. The hair cells of the
organ of Corti initiate impulses via the fibers of the auditory nerve to
the brain.

Quiz: The Sense Organs

1. The inner ear of mammals also contains the apparatus for balance and equilibrium. Changes of the position of the head with respect to gravity, as in bending forward, are detected by hair cells in chambers known as the

   (A)   semicircular canals.

   (B)   vestibular canal.

   (C)   statocyst.

   (D)   utricle and saccule.

   (E)   cochlear duct.

2. The inner ear contains small crystals of calcium carbonate that are involved with the vestibular process of maintaining static equilibrium. These crystals are called

   (A)   otoliths.

   (B)   protostomes.

   (C)   vestibular crystalline apparatus.

   (D)   vestibular clefts.

   (E)   earoliths.

3. Which of the following membranes does a sound wave strike first?

   (A)   Tympanic membrane

   (B)   Membrane of the round window

   (C)   Membrane of the oval window

   (D)   Tectorial membrane

   (E)   None of the above.

4. The sensitivity of the eye to light varies with

   (A) wavelength.

   (B) the eye's state of adaptation.

   (C) the region of the retina.

   (D) the contraction or dilation of the iris.

   (E) All of the above.

5. Receptor cells that are very sensitive to color are the

   (A) ganglion cells.

   (B) rods.

   (C) cones.

   (D) bipolar cells.

   (E) chromatic cells.

6. The colored portion of the eye is called the

   (A) lens.

   (B) cornea.

   (C) pupil.

   (D) iris.

   (E) retina.

7. The retina

   (A) is the round opening in the center of the eye through which light passes.

   (B) is the photosensitive curtain of nerve cells located at the back of the eye.

   (C) bends and focuses light rays.

(D)   protects the internal parts of the eye.

(E)   is the muscle holding the pupil in place.

8.   When light changes from bright to dim, the iris of the eye

(A)   dilates.

(B)   constricts.

(C)   remains the same.

(D)   changes in color.

(E)   thickens.

9.   Eye receptors and their function can best be summarized as

(A)   cones - color discrimination, rods - twilight vision.

(B)   cones - twilight vision, rods - color discrimination.

(C)   ganglia - color discrimination, rods - twilight vision.

(D)   lens - light refraction, cornea - light refraction.

(E)   neurons - twilight vision, ganglia - color discrimination.

10.   The innermost layer of the eye is the

(A)   choroid coat.

(B)   cornea.

(C)   pupil.

(D)   retina.

(E)   sclera.

ANSWER KEY

1.	(D)	6.	(D)
2.	(A)	7.	(B)
3.	(A)	8.	(A)
4.	(E)	9.	(A)
5.	(C)	10.	(D)

CHAPTER 10

The Endocrine System

10.1 Hormone Action

The endocrine system consists of a group of ductless glands that secrete chemical signals, **hormones**, into the bloodstream. As a hormone is transported by the circulating blood, it signals target tissues that respond to this signal. For example, the posterior lobe of the pituitary gland secretes the hormone ADH (antidiuretic hormone). Transported by the blood flow, it reaches the kidney, where its target tissues are found. At this structure it controls water balance.

Chemically, most hormones are either peptides (chains of amino acids) or steroids. Peptide hormones (i.e., insulin) bind to receptors on the cell surfaces at target tissues. This stimulates changes in the metabolism of the cells. One example is an increase in the rate of protein synthesis. Steroid hormones (i.e., aldosterone) bind to receptor molecules in the cytoplasm of the cell that enter the nucleus. In the nucleus they change the genetic activity of the cell.

Hormone signaling influences a wide variety of body functions, ranging from the growth of bones and muscles to the concentration of glucose in the blood.

Problem Solving Example:

Define a hormone. How would you go about proving that a particular gland is responsible for a specific function?

The endocrine system constitutes the second great communicating system of the body, with the first being the nervous system. The endocrine system consists of ductless glands that secrete hormones. A hormone is a chemical substance synthesized by a specific organ or tissue and secreted directly into the blood. The hormone is carried via the circulation to other sites of the body where its actions are exerted. Hormones are typically carried in the blood from the site of production to the site(s) of action, but certain hormones produced by neurosecretory cells in the hypothalamus act directly on their target areas without passing through the blood. The distance travelled by hormones before reaching their target area varies considerably. In terms of chemical structure, hormones generally fall into three categories: The steroid hormones include the sex hormones and the hormones of the adrenal cortex; the amino acid derivatives (of tyrosine) include the thyroid hormones and hormones of the adrenal medulla; proteins and polypeptides make up the majority of the hormones. The chemical structure determines the mechanism of action of the hormone. Hormones serve to control and integrate many body functions such as reproduction, organic metabolism and energy balance, and mineral metabolism. Hormones also regulate a variety of behaviors, including sexual behaviors.

To determine whether a gland is responsible for a particular function or behavior, an investigator usually begins by surgically removing the gland and observing the effect upon the animal. The investigator would then replace the gland with one transplanted from a closely related animal, and determine whether the changes induced by removing the gland can be reversed by replacing it. When replacing the gland, the experimenter must ensure that the new gland becomes connected with the vascular system of the recipient so that secretions from the transplanted gland can enter the blood of the recipient. The experimenter may then try feeding dried glands to an animal from which the gland was previously removed. This is done to see if the hormone can be replaced in the body in this manner. The substance in the glands will enter the bloodstream via the digestive system and be carried to the target organ by the circulatory system. Finally, the experimenter may make an extract of the gland and purify it to determine its chemical structure. Very often the chemical structure of a substance is very much related to its function. Studying the chemical structure may enable the investigator to deduce a mechanism by which the gland extract functions on a molecular level. The investigator may also inject the purified gland extract into an experimental animal devoid of such a gland, and see whether the injection effected replacement of the missing function or behavior. Some hormonal chemicals have additive effects. The investigator may inject a dosage of the purified gland extract to an intact animal to observe if there was any augmentation of the particular function or behavior under study.

10.2 Endocrine Glands

The main endocrine glands are the **pituitary** (anterior and posterior lobes), **thyroid**, **parathyroids**, **adrenal** (cortex and medulla), **pancreas**, and **gonads**.

The pituitary gland is attached to the hypothalamus of the lower forebrain.

The thyroid gland consists of two lateral masses, connected by a crossbridge, that are attached to the trachea. They are slightly inferior to the larynx.

The parathyroids are four masses of tissue, two embedded posteriorly in each lateral mass of the thyroid gland.

One adrenal gland is located on top of each kidney. The cortex is the outer layer of the adrenal gland. The medulla is the inner core.

The pancreas is along the lower curvature of the stomach, close to where it meets the first region of the small intestine, the duodenum.

The gonads are found in the pelvic cavity.

10.3 Pituitary Gland

The pituitary gland consists of the anterior lobe (adenohypophysis) and posterior lobe (neurohypophysis).

Anterior Lobe - Small blood vessels continue from the **hypothalamus** to the endocrine cells of the anterior lobe. **Releasing factors**, chemical signals from the hypothalamus, reach the anterior lobe by the blood flow and influence its activity. Each releasing factor affects the secretion of a hormone from the anterior lobe. For example, **CRF** (corticotropin-releasing factor) signals the anterior lobe to secrete the hormone ACTH (adrenocorticotropic hormone).

Many of the hormones of the anterior lobe are **tropic hormones**. They signal target tissues in other endocrine glands. Tropic hormones include:

ACTH - Signals the adrenal cortex

TSH - Signals the thyroid gland

Gonadotropic hormones - **FSH** in the male and female signals sex cell production and maturation. **LH** in the female signals ovulation. **ICSH** in the male signals the production of testosterone.

There are three related levels of signaling involving the hypothalamus, anterior lobe of the pituitary, and other endocrine glands. One example is:

I.   Hypothalamus secretes a releasing factor, e.g., CRF

II. Anterior lobe of the pituitary secretes a tropic hormone, e.g., ACTH

III. Adrenal cortex secretes cortisol

This response occurs when the level of sugar in the blood decreases. This change is sensed by the hypothalamus. By the three-tiered signaling through the hypothalamus, anterior lobe, and adrenal cortex, the hormone cortisol stimulates a response that increases the level of sugar in the blood. This response reverses the original trend of a decreasing level of sugar in the blood. This pattern of response is an example of **negative feedback** — a response that reverses the trend of the original stimulus.

Some of the hormones secreted by the anterior lobe of the pituitary are not tropic hormones, for they do not signal other endocrine glands. They include:

Growth Hormone (GH, somatotropin) - This stimulates the increase in the use of amino acids, particularly by bones and muscles. During the early years of physical growth, an oversecretion of GH can produce **gigantism**. A deficiency of GH, another imbalance during the years of physical growth, can produce **dwarfism**. An oversecretion of GH later in life produces a condition called **acromegaly**. Only certain bones (e.g., mandible) of the body are affected, leading to the disproportionate growth of body regions.

The growth hormone can also signal many body cells to use fats as a source of energy in preference to glucose. Glucose stays in the blood instead of entering cells as an energy source. Therefore, the growth hormone promotes a hyperglycemic (high blood sugar) effect.

Prolactin - This hormone stimulates the development of mammary glands to produce milk in females.

MSH (melanocyte stimulating hormone) - This hormone may stimulate the skin to increase the production of melanin, a dark pigment found in the skin.

Posterior Lobe - Axons from neurons in the hypothalamus continue into the posterior lobe. The two signals secreted from the posterior lobe are produced by these neurons.

ADH (antidiuretic hormone) - It signals the tubules in the nephrons of the kidney to reabsorb more water. First, water enters the tubules by filtration. By reabsorption it is returned to the blood and, therefore, not eliminated. If the blood lacks sufficient water, the secretion of ADH increases, signaling the kidney to reabsorb more. If the blood has sufficient water, the secretion of ADH and rate of reabsorption decrease. ADH is also called **vasopressin**, as it can constrict blood vessels.

A deficiency of ADH leads to **diabetes insipidus**. Losing some ability to reabsorb water, the person eliminates a large amount of dilute urine.

Oxytocin - It signals the uterus to contract, inducing labor. It also stimulates the release of milk from the breasts when nursing.

Problem Solving Example:

 The pituitary gland has been called the master gland. Is this term justified? Where is the gland located? What does it secrete?

The pituitary gland, also known as the hypophysis, lies in a pocket of bone just below the hypothalamus. The pituitary gland is composed of three lobes, each of which is a functionally distinct gland. They are the anterior, intermediate, and posterior lobes. The anterior and posterior lobes are also known as the adenohypophysis and neurohypophysis, respectively.

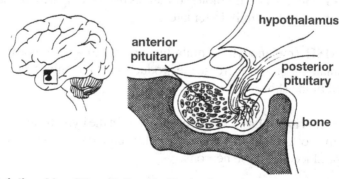

Relationship of the pituitary to the brain and hypothalamus

In humans, the intermediate lobe is only rudimentary and its function remains unclear. It secretes melanocyte stimulating hormone (MSH), which is known to cause skin darkening in the lower vertebrates.

The anterior lobe is made up of glandular tissue, which produces at least six different protein hormones. Evidence suggests that each hormone is secreted by a different cell type. Secretion of each of the six hormones occurs independently of the others.

One of the hormones secreted by the anterior pituitary is known as TSH (thyroid stimulating hormone), which induces secretion of the thyroid hormones from the thyroid gland. Thyroid hormones refer to two closely related hormones, thyroxine (T_4) and triiodothyronine (T_3). Another hormone secreted by the anterior pituitary is ACTH (adrenocorticotropic hormone), which stimulates the adrenal cortex to secrete cortisol. The anterior pituitary is also responsible for the release of the gonadotropic hormones, FSH (follicle stimulating hormone) and LH (luteinizing hormone). These hormones primarily control the secretion of the sex hormones estrogen, progesterone, and testosterone by the gonads. FSH and LH also regulate the growth and development of the reproductive cells (sperm and ovum). TSH, ACTH, FSH, and LH are all tropic hormones in that they stimulate other endocrine glands to secrete hormones. There are two hormones secreted by the anterior pituitary that do not affect other hormonal secretions, but rather act directly on target tissues. One of these is called prolactin, which stimulates milk production by the mammary glands of the female shortly after giving birth. The other hormone is called growth hormone, which plays a critical role in the normal processes of growth.

The posterior lobe of the pituitary gland is actually an outgrowth of the hypothalamus and is neural tissue. The posterior pituitary differs from the anterior pituitary with respect to embryological origin as well as types of hormones secreted. It releases two hormones called oxytocin and vasopressin. Oxytocin principally acts to stimulate contraction of the uterine muscles as an aid to parturition. Emotional stress may also cause the release of this hormone and is frequently the cause of a miscarriage. Oxytocin is also responsible for the milk let-down reflex. It stimulates smooth muscle cells of the mammary glands, which cause milk ejection.

Antidiuretic hormone (ADH) stimulates the kidney tubules to reabsorb water and thus plays an important role in the control of plasma volume. In addition, ADH can increase blood pressure by causing arteriolar constriction. Thus, ADH is also called vasopressin.

It should now be clear why the pituitary is called the master gland; it secretes at least nine hormones, some of which directly regulate life processes while others control the secretion of other glands important in development, behavior, and reproduction.

10.4 Thyroid Gland

The thyroid gland secretes two hormones, **thyroid hormone** and **thyrocalcitonin**.

Thyroid hormone consists of two components, thyroxine and iodine. This hormone increases the rate of metabolism of most body cells. A deficiency of iodine in the diet leads to the enlargement of the thyroid gland, known as a **simple goiter**. Hypothyroidism during early development leads to **cretinism**. In adults, it produces **myxedema**, characterized by obesity and lethargy. Hyperthyroidism leads to a condition called **exophthalmic goiter**, characterized by weight loss as well as hyperactive and irritable behavior.

Thyrocalcitonin (calcitonin) decreases the concentration of calcium in the blood. Most of the calcium removed from the blood is stored in the bones.

Problem Solving Example:

Q The thyroid gland is located in the neck and secretes several hormones, the principal one being thyroxine. Trace the formation of thyroxine. What functions does it serve in the body? What happens when there is a decreased or increased amount of thyroxine in the body?

A The thyroid gland is a two-lobed gland that manifests a remarkably powerful active transport mechanism for the uptake of iodide ions from the blood. As blood flows through the gland, iodide is actively transported into the cells. Once within the cell, the iodide is converted to an active form of iodine. This iodine combines with an amino acid called tyrosine. Two molecules of iodinated tyrosine then combine to form thyroxine. Following its formation, the thyroxine becomes bound to a polysaccharide-protein material called thyroglobulin. The normal thyroid gland may store several weeks' supply of thyroxine in this bound form. An enzymatic splitting of the thyroxine from the thyroglobulin occurs when a specific hormone is released into the blood. This hormone, produced by the pituitary gland, is known as thyroid-stimulating hormone (TSH). TSH stimulates certain major rate-limiting steps in thyroxine secretion, and thereby alters its rate of release. A variety of bodily defects, either dietary, hereditary, or disease-induced, may decrease the amount of thyroxine released into the blood. The most popular of these defects is one that results from dietary iodine deficiency. The thyroid gland enlarges, in the continued presence of TSH from the pituitary, to form a goiter. This is a futile attempt to synthesize thyroid hormones, for iodine levels are low. Normally, thyroid hormones act via a negative feedback loop on the pituitary to decrease stimulation of the thyroid. In goiter, the feedback loop cannot be in operation — hence continual stimulation of the thyroid and the inevitable protuberance on the neck. Formerly, the principal source of iodine came from seafood. As a result, goiter was prevalent amongst inland areas far removed from the sea. Today, the incidence of goiter has been drastically reduced by adding iodine to table salt.

Thyroxine serves to stimulate oxidative metabolism in cells; it increases the oxygen consumption and heat production of most body tissues, a notable exception being the brain. Thyroxine is also necessary for normal growth, the most likely explanation being that thyroxine promotes the effects of growth hormone on protein synthesis. The absence of thyroxine significantly reduces the ability of growth hormone to stimulate amino acid uptake and RNA synthesis. Thyroxine also plays a crucial role in the closely related area of organ development, particularly that of the central nervous system.

If there is an insufficient amount of thyroxine, a condition referred to as hypothyroidism results. Symptoms of hypothyroidism stem from the fact that there is a reduction in the rate of oxidative energy-releasing reactions within the body cells. Usually the patient shows puffy skin, sluggishness, and lowered vitality. Hypothyroidism in children, a condition known as cretinism, can result in mental retardation, dwarfism, and permanent sexual immaturity. Sometimes the thyroid gland produces too much thyroxine, a condition known as hyperthyroidism. This condition produces symptoms such as an abnormally high body temperature, profuse sweating, high blood pressure, loss of weight, irritability, and muscular weakness. It also produces one very characteristic symptom that may not be predicted because it lacks an obvious connection to a high metabolic rate. This symptom is exophthalmia, a condition where the eyeballs protrude in a startling manner. Hyperthyroidism has been treated by partial removal or by partial radiation destruction of the gland. More recently, several drugs that inhibit thyroid activity have been discovered, and their use is supplanting the former surgical procedures.

10.5 Parathyroid Glands

The four parathyroids secrete the **parathyroid hormone** (PTH). It opposes the effect of thyrocalcitonin. It does this by removing calcium from its storage sites in bones, releasing it into the bloodstream. It also signals the kidneys to reabsorb more of this mineral, transporting it into the blood. It also signals the small intestine to absorb more of this mineral, transporting it from the diet into the blood.

Calcium is important for many steps of body metabolism. Blood cannot clot without sufficient calcium. Skeletal muscles require this mineral in order to contract. A deficiency of PTH can lead to **tetany**, muscle weakness due to a lack of available calcium in the blood.

Problem Solving Example:

Q The parathyroid glands in humans are small, pea-like organs. They are usually four in number and are located on the surface of the thyroid. What is the function of these glands?

A The parathyroids were long thought to be part of the thyroid or to be functionally associated with it. Now, however, we know that their close proximity to the thyroid is misleading; both developmentally and functionally, they are totally distinct from the thyroid.

The parathyroid hormone, called parathormone, regulates the calcium-phosphate balance between the blood and other tissues. Production of this hormone is directly controlled by the calcium concentration of the extracellular fluid bathing the cells of these glands. Parathormone exerts at least the following four effects: (1) it increases gastrointestinal absorption of calcium by stimulating the active-transport system and moves calcium from the gut lumen into the blood; (2) it increases the movement of calcium and phosphate from bone into extracellular fluid. This is accomplished by stimulating osteoclasts to break down bone structure, thus liberating calcium phosphate into the blood. In this way, the store of calcium contained in bone is tapped; (3) it increases reabsorption of calcium by the renal tubules, thereby decreasing urinary calcium excretion; and (4) it reduces the reabsorption of phosphate by the renal tubules.

The first three effects result in a higher extracellular calcium concentration. The adaptive value of the fourth is to prevent the formation of kidney stones.

Should the parathyroids be removed accidentally during surgery on the thyroid, there would be a rise in the phosphate concentration in the blood. There would also be a drop in the calcium concentration as more calcium is excreted by the kidneys and intestines, and more is incorporated into bone. This can produce serious disturbances, particularly in the muscles and nerves, which use calcium ions for normal functioning. Overactivity of the parathyroids, which can result from a tumor on the glands, produces a weakening of the bones. This is a condition that makes them much more vulnerable to fracturing because of excessive withdrawal of calcium from the bones.

10.6 Adrenal Glands

The adrenal **cortex** secretes at least two families of hormones, the **glucocorticoids** and **mineralocorticoids**. The adrenal **medulla** secretes the hormones **epinephrine** (adrenalin) and **norepinephrine** (noradrenalin).

Cortisol is one of the most active glucocorticoids. It generally reduces the effects of inflammation (i.e., swelling) throughout the body. It also stimulates the production of glucose from fats and proteins. This process is called **gluconeogenesis**.

Aldosterone is one example of a mineralocorticoid. It signals the tubules in the kidney nephrons to reabsorb sodium while secreting (eliminating) potassium. If sodium levels are low in the blood, the kidney secretes more **renin**, an enzyme that stimulates the formation of **angiotensin** from a molecule made from the liver. Angiotensin stimulates aldosterone secretion. As a result, more sodium is reabsorbed as it enters the blood.

The renin-angiotensin-aldosterone mechanism can raise blood pressure if it tends to drop. It does this two ways. Angiotensin is a vasoconstrictor, decreasing the diameter of blood vessels. As vessels constrict, blood pressure increases. In addition, as sodium is reabsorbed, the blood passing through the kidney becomes more hypertonic. Water follows the sodium into the hypertonic blood by osmosis. This increases the amount of volume in the blood and also increases blood pressure.

An oversecretion of the glucocorticoids causes **Cushing's syndrome**, characterized by muscle atrophy (degeneration) and hypertension (high blood pressure). A deficiency of these substances produces **Addison's disease**, characterized by low blood pressure and the development of stress.

Epinephrine and norepinephrine produce the "fight-or-flight" response, similar to the effect from the sympathetic nervous system. Therefore, they increase heart rate, breathing rate, blood flow to most skeletal muscles, and the concentration of glucose in the blood. They decrease the blood flow to digestive organs and diminish most digestive processes.

Problem Solving Examples:

Q The cortex of the adrenal gland is known to produce over 20 hormones, but their study can be simplified by classifying them into three categories: glucocorticoids, mineralocorticoids, and sex hormones. Explain the function and give examples of each of these three groups of hormones. What will result from a hypofunctional adrenal cortex?

A The glucocorticoids include corticosterone, cortisone, and hydrocortisone (cortisol). These hormones serve to stimulate the conversion of amino acids into carbohydrates (a process known as gluconeogenesis) and the formation of glycogen by the liver. They also stimulate formation of reserve glycogen in the tissues, such as in muscles. The glucocorticoids also participate in lipid and protein metabolism. Glucocorticoids are also essential for coping with stress and acting as anti-inflammatory agents. Glucocorticoid secretion is controlled by the anterior pituitary hormone ACTH (adrenocorticotropic hormone).

Aldosterone, the major mineralocorticoid, stimulates the cells of the distal convoluted tubules of the kidneys to decrease reabsorption of potassium and increase reabsorption of sodium. This in turn leads to an increased reabsorption of chloride and water. These hormones, together with such hormones as insulin and glucagon, are important regulators of the ionic environment of the internal fluid.

The adrenal sex hormones consist mainly of male sex hormones (androgens) and lesser amounts of female sex hormones (estrogens and progesterone). Normally, the sex hormones released from the adrenal cortex are insignificant due to the low concentration of secretion. However, in cases of excess secretion, masculinizing or feminizing effects appear. The most common syndrome of this sort is virilism of the female.

Should there be an insufficient supply of cortical hormones, a condition known as Addison's disease would result. This disease is characterized by an excessive excretion of sodium ions, and hence water, due to a lack of mineralocorticoids. Accompanying this is a decreased blood glucose level due to a deficient supply of glucocorticoids. The effect of a decreased androgen supply cannot be observed immediately. Injections of adrenal cortical hormones promptly relieve these symptoms.

Hormonal production in the adrenal cortex is directly controlled by the anterior pituitary hormone called adrenocorticotropic hormone (ACTH).

Q The two adrenal glands lie very close to the kidneys. Each adrenal gland is actually a double gland, composed of an inner corelike medulla and an outer cortex. Each of these is functionally unrelated. Outline the function of the adrenal medulla.

A The adrenal medulla secretes two hormones, adrenalin (epinephrine) and noradrenalin (norepinephrine), whose functions are very similar but not identical. The adrenal medulla is derived embryologically from neural tissue. It has been likened to an overgrown sympathetic ganglion whose cell bodies do not send out nerve fibers, but release their active substances directly into the blood, thereby fulfilling the criteria for an endocrine gland. In controlling epinephrine secretion, the adrenal medulla behaves just like any sympathetic ganglion, and is dependent upon stimulation by sympathetic preganglionic fibers, as shown below:

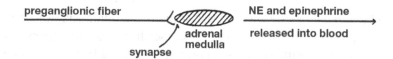

preganglionic fiber

NE and epinephrine released into blood

adrenal medulla

synapse

Epinephrine promotes several responses, all of which are helpful in coping with emergencies: the blood pressure rises, the heart rate increases, the glucose content of the blood rises because of glycogen breakdown, the spleen contracts and squeezes out a reserve supply of blood, the clotting time of blood decreases, the pupils dilate, the blood flow to skeletal muscle increases, the blood supply to intestinal smooth muscle decreases, and hairs become erect. These adrenal functions, which mobilize the resources of the body in emergencies, have been called the fight-or-flight response. Norepinephrine stimulates reactions similar to those produced by epinephrine, but is less effective in the conversion of glycogen into glucose.

The significance of the adrenal medulla may seem questionable since the complete removal of the gland causes few noticeable changes; humans can still exhibit the fight-or-flight response. This occurs because the sympathetic nervous system complements the adrenal medulla in stimulating the fight-or-flight response, and the absence of the hormonal control will be compensated for by the nervous system.

10.7 Pancreas

The pancreas contains exocrine and endocrine cells. Groups of endocrine cells, the **islets of Langerhans**, secrete two hormones. The beta cells secrete **insulin**; the alpha cells secrete **glucagon**. The level of sugar in the blood depends on the opposing action of these two hormones.

Insulin decreases the concentration of glucose in the blood. Most of the glucose enters the cells of the liver and skeletal muscles. In these cells this monosaccharide is converted to the polysaccharide glycogen. Therefore, insulin promotes **glycogenesis**, glycogen formation.

Glucagon promotes **glycogenolysis**, the breakdown of glycogen into glucose for release into the blood.

Insulin deficiency leads to the development of **diabetes mellitus**, specifically **type I** (juvenile) diabetes. As the pancreas does not produce sufficient insulin, this disorder is treated by insulin injections. In **type II** (maturity onset) diabetes, the pancreas does produce enough insulin, but the target cells do not respond to it.

Problem Solving Example:

Q The pancreas is a mixed gland having both endocrine and exocrine functions. The exocrine portion secretes digestive enzymes into the duodenum via the pancreatic duct. The endocrine portion secretes two hormones (insulin and glucagon) into the blood. What are the effects of these two hormones?

A Insulin is a hormone that acts directly or indirectly on most tissues of the body, with the exception of the brain. The most important action of insulin is the stimulation of the uptake of glucose by many tissues, particularly the liver, muscle, and fat. The uptake of glucose by the cells decreases blood glucose and increases the availability of glucose for those cellular reactions in which glucose participates. Thus, glucose oxidation, fat synthesis, and glycogen synthesis are all accentuated by an uptake of glucose. It is important to note that insulin does not alter glucose uptake by the brain, nor does it influence the active transport of glucose across the renal tubules and gastrointestinal epithelium.

As stated, insulin stimulates glycogen synthesis. In addition, it also increases the activity of the enzyme that catalyzes the rate-limiting step in glycogen synthesis. Insulin also increases triglyceride levels by inhibiting triglyceride breakdown, and by stimulating production of triglyceride through fatty acid and glycerophosphate synthesis. The net protein synthesis is also increased by insulin, which stimulates the active membrane transport of amino acids, particularly into muscle cells. Insulin also has effects on other liver enzymes, but the precise mechanisms by which insulin induces these changes are poorly understood.

Insulin secretion is directly controlled by the glucose concentration of the blood flowing through the pancreas. This is a simple system that requires no participation of nerves or other hormones.

Insulin is secreted by beta cells, which are located in the part of the pancreas known as the islets of Langerhans. These groups of cells, which are located randomly throughout the pancreas, also consist of other secretory cells called alpha cells. It is these alpha cells that secrete glucagon. Glucagon is a hormone that has the following major effects: it increases glycogen breakdown, thereby raising the plasma glucose level; it increases hepatic synthesis of glucose from pyruvate, lactate, glycerol, and amino acids (a process called gluconeogenesis, which also raises the plasma glucose level); and it increases the breakdown of adipose-tissue triglyceride, thereby raising the plasma levels of fatty acids and glycerol. The glucagon-secreting alpha cells in the pancreas, like the beta cells, respond to changes in the concentration of glucose in the blood flowing through the pancreas; no other nerves or hormones are involved.

It should be noted that glucagon has the opposite effects of insulin. Glucagon elevates the plasma glucose, whereas insulin stimulates its uptake and thereby reduces plasma glucose levels; glucagon elevates fatty acid concentrations, whereas insulin converts fatty acids (and glycerol) into triglycerides, thereby inhibiting triglyceride breakdown.

Thus, the alpha and beta cells of the pancreas constitute a "push-pull" system for regulating the plasma glucose level.

10.8 Gonads

The main hormones from the reproductive organs are:

Testosterone - This hormone is more prominent in males. It belongs to the family of androgens, which are steroid hormones producing masculinizing effects. Testosterone stimulates the development and functioning of the primary sex organs. It also stimulates the development and maintenance of secondary male characteristics, such as hair growth on the face and the deep pitch of the voice.

Estrogen - In females, this hormone stimulates the development of the uterus and vagina. It is also responsible for the development and maintenance of secondary female characteristics, such as fat distribution throughout the body and the width of the pelvis.

Progesterone - In females this hormone also stimulates development of primary and secondary female characteristics. Known as the hormone of pregnancy, it is very prominent in the last 14 days of the female reproductive cycle, occurring after ovulation. One of its effects is to increase the thickness and development of the uterine lining for implantation of an embryo if fertilization occurs.

Problem Solving Example:

 What hormones are involved with the changes that occur in pubescent females and males?

Puberty begins in the female when the hypothalamus stimulates the anterior pituitary to release increased amounts of FSH (follicle stimulating hormone) and LH (luteinizing hormone). These hormones cause the ovaries to mature and to begin secreting estrogen and progesterone, the female sex hormones. These hormones, particularly estrogen, are responsible for the development of the female secondary sexual characteristics. These characteristics include the growth of pubic hair, an increase in the size of the uterus and vagina, a broadening of the hips and development of the breasts, a change in voice quality, and the onset of the menstrual cycle.

Before the onset of puberty in the male, no sperm and very little male sex hormone are produced by the testes. The onset of puberty begins, as in the female, when the hypothalamus stimulates the anterior pituitary to release increased amounts of FSH and LH. In the male, FSH stimulates maturation of the seminiferous tubules, which produce the sperm. LH is responsible for the maturation of the interstitial cells of the testes. It also induces them to begin secretion of testosterone, the male sex hormone. When enough testosterone accumulates, it brings about the whole spectrum of secondary sexual characteristics normally associated with puberty. These include growth of facial and pubic hair, deepening of the voice, maturation of the seminal vesicles and the prostate gland, broadening of the shoulders, and the development of the muscles. If the testes were removed before puberty, the secondary sexual characteristics would fail to develop. If they were removed after puberty, there would be some retrogression of the adult sexual characteristics, but they would not disappear entirely.

10.9 Other Hormones and Endocrine Glands

Endocrinology is a rapidly expanding field, with new endocrine structures and hormones being discovered on a regular basis. Other well-known hormones, in addition to the main ones recognized in this chapter, include:

Erythropoietin - Secreted from endocrine cells in the kidney, it stimulates erythropoiesis (red blood cell formation).

Gastrin - Secreted from endocrine cells in the stomach, it stimulates increased gastric secretions from this organ.

Secretin - Secreted from endocrine cells of the small intestine, it stimulates increased secretions from the pancreas into the small intestine.

Prostaglandins - This is a group of local hormones throughout the body that act close to their site of secretion. Their functions range from influences on blood clotting to effects on inflammation.

Quiz: The Endocrine System

1. Which gland releases GH (growth hormone)?

    (A) Anterior pituitary   (D) Adrenal cortex

    (B) Posterior pituitary   (E) Thyroid

    (C) Adrenal medulla

2.   In males, which of the following hormones is responsible for secondary sexual characteristics?

   (A) Estrogen

   (B) Progesterone

   (C) Growth hormone

   (D) Prolactin

   (E) Testosterone

3.   Excision of the parathyroid glands would result in

   (A) muscle convulsions.

   (B) strengthening of muscles.

   (C) weakening of bones.

   (D) decalcification of bones.

   (E) hypermobility.

4.   The pituitary regulates all of the following except the

   (A) thyroid.   (D) testes.

   (B) adrenal cortex.   (E) adrenal medulla.

   (C) ovaries.

5.   The posterior lobe of the pituitary gland in humans releases

   (A) TSH and FSH.

   (B) ACTH and LH.

   (C) oxytocin and vasopressin.

   (D) FSH and LH.

   (E) prolactin and growth hormone.

6. Which of the following has direct control over the function of the pituitary gland?

    (A) Pons   (D) Midbrain

    (B) Cerebral cortex   (E) Cerebellum

    (C) Hypothalamus

7. Which of the following effects does epinephrine have on the body?

    (A) Constriction of the pupils

    (B) Increased rate of digestion

    (C) Accelerated heartbeat

    (D) Increased hormone production

    (E) Decreased hormone production

8. The pituitary gland secretes which of the following hormones?

    (A) TSH (thyroid stimulating hormone)

    (B) ACTH (adrenocorticotropic hormone)

    (C) FSH (follicle stimulating hormone)

    (D) LH (luteinizing hormone)

    (E) All of the above.

9. The mineral necessary for thyroxine synthesis is

    (A) Ca.

    (B) Fe.

    (C) I.

    (D) P.

    (E) S.

10. The effect of which of the following hormones opposes the effects of the other four?

    (A) Cortisol

    (B) Epinephrine

    (C) Glucagon

    (D) Growth hormone

    (E) Insulin

ANSWER KEY

1.	(A)	6.	(C)
2.	(E)	7.	(C)
3.	(A)	8.	(E)
4.	(E)	9.	(C)
5.	(C)	10.	(E)

CHAPTER 11

The Circulatory System

11.1 Functions

The circulatory system consists of the **blood, heart,** and **blood vessels**. The heart functions as a pump, forcing blood through a series of vessels that distribute the blood to the cells of all body regions. The blood offers oxygen and substances necessary for cell metabolism. The blood also removes waste products from these cells. As the blood carries out this role of internal transport, it travels to and from the various body regions it serves. In other words, it circulates.

The circulatory system meets other needs of body metabolism. Buffers in the blood are substances that stabilize the pH of the fluid surrounding cells (extracellular fluid). By the dilation and constriction of blood vessels in the skin, heat from the body can be either liberated or conserved. This response contributes to the control of internal body temperature.

The circulatory system is also part of the body's immune system. White blood cells (leukocytes) act as a main line of defense that fights infection. In addition, the circulating blood is a vehicle for transporting hormones from endocrine glands to target tissues.

11.2 Blood

The adult human body contains an average of five liters of blood. Blood consists of three kinds of specialized cells (formed elements): **erythrocytes** (red blood cells), **leukocytes** (white blood cells), and **thrombocytes** (platelets). As the blood circulates, these cells are suspended in a liquid matrix, the **plasma**. Normally, the cells make up about 45 percent of the blood by volume (see figure below). The blood can also be typed into four classes (ABO bloodtyping).

The percentage of the blood that is cellular by volume is called the **hematocrit**. This can be measured and computed by laboratory tests. The cells in a test-tube sample of blood can be packed into the bottom of the tube. The plasma, which is not as dense as the cells, settles above the cells in the test tube. If, for example, the cells make up 9 volume units in a total of 20 units of blood, the hematocrit is 45 percent. The plasma in this case composes the other 55 percent.

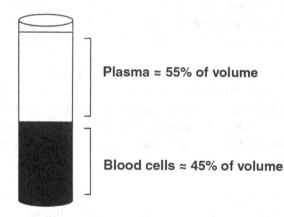

Plasma ≈ 55% of volume

Blood cells ≈ 45% of volume

Test tube of blood cells and plasma

Erythrocytes - Erythrocytes are the gas carriers of the blood. They are small, biconcave disks. At maturity they lack a nucleus and the organelles common to most cells. They do, however, contain millions of molecules of **hemoglobin**. This pigment has the ability to combine reversibly with oxygen. Oxygen combines with hemoglobin, forming oxyhemoglobin as blood passes through the lungs. It dissociates from hemoglobin at tissue sites throughout the body, releasing it for use by cell metabolism.

The hemoglobin in erythrocytes also transports carbon dioxide. It receives carbon dioxide from cells as a product of their metabolism, then unloads it at the lungs for elimination from the body.

Erythrocytes, along with leukocytes and thrombocytes, can be counted on a per cubic millimeter (mm) basis. A normal count ranges from about 4.2 million to 6 million per cubic millimeter. The count is usually somewhat higher in males than in females. An abnormally low red cell count and/or hemoglobin deficiency produces **anemia**, the inability of the blood to carry and deliver sufficient oxygen to the body cells.

Erythrocytes are produced from the red bone marrow in the ends of long bones, cranial bones, ribs, sternum, and vertebrae. The early stages of red cells have a nucleus. Lacking a nucleus by the time they are released into the circulation, they cannot reproduce. A normal life span for a red blood cell is 120 days.

Eventually, red blood cells are destroyed by phagocytic cells in the liver and spleen. The hemo portion of the hemoglobin molecule, which contains iron, is sent to the liver for reuse by the body. The globin portion, a protein, is converted into bile in the liver by a series of steps. Stored in the gallbladder, bile is secreted into the small intestine for the physical digestion of fats in the diet.

Leukocytes - Leukocytes have a nucleus and are larger than erythrocytes. Most of them are produced in the bone marrow. A **total** white blood cell **count** normally ranges from 5,000 to 10,000 per cubic millimeter. **Leukopenia** is revealed by a white cell count that is less than the lower end of this range. Leukocytosis is a high white cell count, above 10,000 per cubic millimeter.

There are five different kinds of white blood cells. Each kind makes up a percentage of the total white cell count. White blood cells lack pigments. They can be stained and examined under the microscope in order to be distinguished from each other. Each kind of white cell has unique characteristics revealed through this procedure.

Three kinds of leukocytes contain stained granules in the cytoplasm: **neutrophil**, **basophil**, and **eosinophil**. Two kinds lack granules: **lymphocyte** and **monocyte**. The neutrophil, for example, has a nucleus with many interconnected lobes and blue granules. By contrast, the nucleus of the eosinophil lacks lobes, but it has reddish-orange granules.

In addition to the total count, a **differential** white cell **count** can also be conducted on white blood cells. This charts the percentage of each kind of cell in the total count. Neutrophils, for example, make up around 65 percent of the total count; lymphocytes make up about 25 percent. Information from a differential count can have diagnostic value. If, for example, the percentage of eosinophils increases, it usually means the body has an allergy.

Leukocytes fight infection in several ways. Some are phagocytic, capable of engulfing foreign cells such as invading bacteria. They can leave the circulation and enter the intercellular spaces to do this, an action called **diapedesis**. Lymphocytes can produce molecules, called **antibodies**, that react against foreign substances, **antigens**, entering the body reacting with them and destroying them.

Thrombocytes - These platelets are cell fragments, produced from large cells, megakaryocytes, in the bone marrow. A normal platelet count ranges from 200,000 to 400,000 per cubic millimeter.

Platelets initiate the process of blood clotting. They are attracted to a rough texture on the inside surface of a blood vessel. Normally this surface is smooth, but can be changed by a cut or deposit (e.g., cholesterol).

If platelets are attracted to a rough surface, platelets release a group of substances called platelet factors (thromboplastins). These factors react through a series of chemical changes, leading to the conversion of fibrinogen to **fibrin**. Fibrinogen is a plasma protein. Fibrin is an insoluble protein that traps red blood cells, forming a clot. This clot can plug vessels, preventing blood from escaping.

Plasma - As the liquid portion of the blood, the plasma is 90 to 92 percent water. Many kinds of substances are dissolved or suspended in this medium. Some are nutrients from the diet: glucose and amino acids. Others are waste products: lactic acid and urea (for nitrogen elimination). Other substances include minerals, hormones, and antibodies. All of these substances are part of body metabolism.

Blood Typing - The most common blood typing system is the **ABO** system, which depends on the presence or absence of two **antigens**, A and B. If only one is present on the surface of the erythrocytes, the blood type is either **A** or **B**. If both are present, the blood type is **AB**. If neither is present, the type is **O**, the most common ABO blood type. Therefore, the antigen content names the blood type.

Two **antibodies**, anti-A and anti-B, are present in the plasma and are also part of the ABO system. This antibody makeup is normally the opposite, by letter, of the antigen in a person's blood. For example, if a person has only the A antigen (type A), anti-B is present in the person's plasma. A type B person (B antigen) has the anti-A antibody. A type AB person (both antigens) has neither antibody. A type O person has both antibodies.

An **agglutination** (clotting) reaction occurs if the antigen and antibody of the same letter are mixed. Although this does not normally occur in a person's own blood, it can occur through a mistake of blood transfusion. If type A blood is transfused into a person with type B blood (anti-A antibodies present), the two blood types will clot, leading to the death of the individual receiving the blood.

11.3 Heart – Structure and Function

The heart works as a double pump. The right side pumps blood to the lungs; the left side sends the blood to all other body locations. The adult heart is about the size of a closed fist. About two-thirds of its mass is to the left of the body midline. Residing in the mediastinum, the heart is housed in a loose-fitting sac, the **pericardium**. Its apex, the cone-shaped inferior portion, fits into a depression on the diaphragm.

The anatomy of the heart consists of chambers, associated blood vessels, valves, and a conduction system.

Chambers - The **atria** (singular, atrium) are the two superior chambers of the heart. A **ventricle** is inferior to each atrium on each side of the heart. The ventricles are larger chambers with thicker muscular walls (cardiac muscle tissue). The left ventricle is the most powerful pumping chamber of the heart. A septum (wall) separates the right atrium from the left atrium. It also separates the two ventricles.

The muscle wall of each chamber, the **myocardium**, is lined internally by the **endocardium**, a layer of epithelium.

Associated Blood Vessels - Several major blood vessels connect to the heart, transporting blood to and from this organ. Each vessel is either an artery or a vein. **Arteries** transport blood away from the heart. **Veins** return blood to the heart.

The **superior** and **inferior vena cava** are the two thickest veins of the body. The superior vena cava drains blood from the head, neck, and arms into the right atrium. As the second longest vein of the body, the inferior vena cava transports blood into the right atrium from all other body regions.

The **pulmonary trunk** transports blood from the right ventricle. Dividing into a right and left **pulmonary artery**, the blood flow continues to the lungs.

Four **pulmonary veins**, two from each lung, return blood to the left atrium.

The **aorta**, the largest artery in the body, transports blood from the left ventricle, priming the arteries that serve all body regions except the lungs. Shortly after the aorta exits from the left ventricle, two **coronary arteries** send some blood back to the heart tissues. This blood supplies the heart cells with their necessary oxygen and nutrients.

Valves - There are two pairs of valves in the heart. The **AV** (atrioventricular) **valves** are found between the atria and ventricles. Also called the cuspid valves, the **bicuspid** valve (mitral valve) is between the atrium and ventricle on the left. The **tricuspid** valve is between these chambers on the right.

The semilunar valves (half-moon shaped) are located where the major artery exits from the ventricle on each side. The **pulmonary semilunar valve** is located where the pulmonary trunk exits from the right ventricle. The **aortic semilunar valve** is located where the aorta exits from the left ventricle.

Valves can open and close. When closed, they prevent the backflow of blood. On each side the blood flows from the atrium to the ventricle through the outgoing artery. The AV (cuspid) valves close to prevent the backflow of blood to the atria. Each AV valve is attached to the **chordae tendinae**. These string-like structures are anchored to the **papillary muscles**, elevated masses of muscle tissue in the ventricles.

The semilunar valves close to prevent the backflow of blood to the ventricles, sealing off this possibility and ensuring that blood flows through the pulmonary trunk and aorta instead.

Problem Solving Example:

 Trace the path of blood through the human heart.

 The heart is the muscular organ that causes blood to circulate in the body. The heart is a pulsatile four-chambered pump composed of an upper left and right atrium (plural, atria) and a lower left and right ventricle. The atria function mainly as entryways to the ventricles, whereas the ventricles supply the main force that propels blood to the lungs and throughout the body.

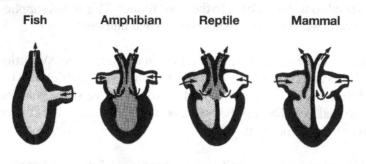

The hearts of four classes of vertebrates. From fish to mammal, there is increasing separation between the two sides of the heart, with consequent decrease in the amount of mixing between oxygenated and deoxygenated blood.

Depending on where the blood is flowing from, it enters the heart via one of the two veins: the superior vena cava carries blood from the head, neck, and arms; the inferior vena cava carries blood from the rest of the body. The blood from these two veins enters the right atrium. When this chamber is filled with blood, the chamber contracts and forces the blood through a valve called the tricuspid valve and into the right ventricle. Since this blood has returned from its circulation in the body's tissues, it is deoxygenated and contains much carbon dioxide. It therefore must be transported to the lungs where gas exchange can take place. The right ventricle contracts, forces the blood through the pulmonary semilunar valve and into the pulmonary artery. This artery is unlike most arteries in that it carries deoxygenated blood. The artery splits into two, with one branch leading to each lung. The pulmonary arteries further divide into many arterioles, which divide even further and connect with dense capillary networks surrounding the alveoli in the lungs. The alveoli are small sac-like cavities where gas exchange occurs. Carbon dioxide diffuses into the alveoli, where it is expelled, while oxygen is picked up by the hemoglobin of the erythrocytes. The capillaries join to form small venules, which further combine to form the four pulmonary veins leading back to the heart. The pulmonary veins are unlike most veins in that they carry oxygenated blood.

These veins empty into the left atrium, which contracts to force the blood through the bicuspid (or mitral) valve and into the left ventricle. When the left ventricle, filled with blood, contracts, the blood is forced though the aortic semilunar valve into the aorta, the largest artery in the body (about 25 mm in diameter).

The aorta forms an arch and runs posteriorly and inferiorly along the body. Before it completes the arch, the aorta branches into the coronary artery, which carries blood to the muscular walls of the heart itself, the carotid arteries, which carry blood to the head and brain, and the subclavian arteries, which carry blood to the arms. As the aorta runs posteriorly, it branches into arteries that lead to various organs such as the liver, kidney, intestines, spleen, and the legs.

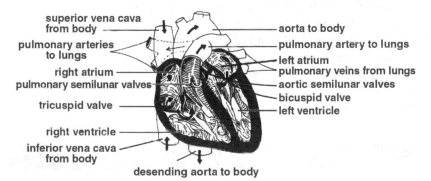

Diagram of the human heart showing chambers, valves, and connecting vessels

The arteries divide into arterioles, which further divide and become capillaries. It is here that the oxygen and nutrients diffuse into the tissues and carbon dioxide and nitrogenous wastes are picked up. The capillaries fuse to form venules, which further fuse to become either the superior or inferior vena cava. The entire cycle starts once again.

The part of the circulatory system in which deoxygenated blood is pumped to the lungs and oxygenated blood returned to the heart is called the pulmonary circulation. The part in which oxygenated blood is pumped to all parts of the body by the arteries and deoxygenated blood is returned to the heart by the veins is called the systemic circulation.

Conduction System - The heart contains masses of nodal tissue, excitable tissue that conducts impulses and stimulates the heartbeat intrinsically. This conduction system signals the heart to beat independently. It does not require any external influences. The impulse to stimulate the heartbeat passes through the conduction system structures in this order: **SA node - AV node - AV bundle - Purkinje fibers**.

The SA (sinoatrial) node, known as the pacemaker, is in the wall of the right atrium, near the entrance of the superior vena cava. By initiating the impulse for each heartbeat, the SA node sends an impulse through the myocardium of both atria, depolarizing the muscle cells of these chambers. This causes atrial contraction.

The AV (atrioventricular) node at the base of the right atrium receives an impulse from the walls of the atrium, relaying it through the left and right bundle branches of the AV bundle (bundle of His), located in the septum between the two ventricles. At the apex of the heart, these two branches subdivide into numerous Purkinje fibers. These fibers deliver impulses to the myocardial cells in the ventricles, depolarizing them for contraction.

Problem Solving Example:

Q The heart is removed from the body and placed in an isosmotic solution. Although it is completely separated from nerves, it continues to beat. Explain.

A The initiation of the heartbeat and the beat itself are intrinsic properties of the heart and are not dependent upon stimulation from the central nervous system. The heart is stimulated by two sets of nerves (the sympathetic and vagus nerves), but these only partly regulate the rate of the beat, and are not responsible for the beat itself.

The initiation of the heartbeat originates from a small strip of specialized muscle in the wall of the right atrium called the sino-atrial (SA) node, which is also called the pacemaker of the heart. It is the SA node that generates the rhythmic self-excitatory impulse, causing a wave of contraction across the walls of the atria (see figure below). This wave of contraction reaches a second mass of nodal muscle called the atrioventricular node, or AV node. The atrioventricular node is found in the lower part of the interatrial septum. As the wave of contraction reaches the AV node, the wave stimulates the node, which produces an excitatory impulse. This impulse is rapidly transmitted to a bundle of nodal fibers called the AV bundle or bundle of His. This bundle divides into right and left bundle branches that deliver the impulse to the ventricular myocardium (the muscular layer of the heart wall) via the Purkinje fibers. The impulse is then transmitted to all parts of the ventricles, causing them to contract as a unit.

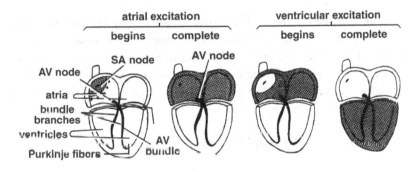

Sequence of cardiac excitation

As the cardiac impulse travels from the SA node through the atria, the wave of contraction forces blood through the valves and into the ventricles. (In the atria, the impulse is transmitted from cell to cell across the intercalated discs.) It is a "wave" of contraction because parts of the atria farthest from the SA node contract later than do the parts closest to the node. The parts of the atria that contract first are also the first to relax, thus causing a wave-like motion upon contraction. Once the impulse reaches the AV node, it is delayed (by a fraction of a second) before it is passed on to the ventricles. This transmission delay allows time for the atria to pump the blood into the ventricles before ventricular contraction begins. Unlike the atria, the ventricles contract as a unit because of the rapid transmission of the impulse by the Purkinje fibers. For example, in the atria, the impulse travels at a velocity of 0.3 meters per second, whereas in the Purkinje fibers, the impulse travels at about 2 meters per second. This allows almost immediate transmission of the impulse throughout the ventricular system.

The adaptive significance of the contraction of the ventricles as a unit rather than as a wave is clear. The ventricles (especially the left ventricle) must exert as great a pressure as possible in order to force the blood through a long system of arteries, capillaries, and veins. A greater pressure is more easily obtained if the ventricles contract as a unit, rather than in waves.

11.3.1 Cardiac Cycle

The cardiac cycle is a repeating series of events that take place each time the heart beats. These events include the **systole** (contraction) and **diastole** (relaxation) of the heart chambers. The two sides of the heart do not contract independently but respond in unison. If we consider an average cycle to require 0.8 seconds, the events can be summarized in three steps.

1. atria, systole; ventricles, diastole (first 0.1 s)

2. atria, diastole; ventricles, systole (next 0.3 s)

3. atria, diastole; ventricles, diastole (last 0.4 s)

First, as the atria contract, the ventricles relax. As the ventricles contract, the atria relax. For the last half of the cycle, all chambers are relaxed.

Cardiac output is the total volume of blood pumped from the left ventricle through the aorta each minute. It is the product of the **heart rate** and **stroke volume**. For example, if the heart beats 70 times per minute and ejects 80 ml of blood per beat (stroke volume), the cardiac output is:

$$70 \times 80 \text{ ml} = 5,600 \text{ ml or } 5.6 \text{ liters}$$

The **ECG** (EKG), electrocardiogram, is a recording of the electrical activity of the heart, accounting for the events of the cycle. The ECG consists of the following waves, recorded in this order for each cardiac cycle:

P wave - From depolarization of the atria—this electrical change produces atrial systole.

QRS complex - From the depolarization of the ventricles—this change produces ventricular systole. The atria are experiencing diastole at this time, but it is not recorded.

T wave - From the repolarization of the ventricles—this change produces ventricular diastole.

Problem Solving Example:

Q When the atria contract, only 30 percent of the ventricular space becomes filled. How does the additional 70 percent become filled? Describe the process of the cardiac cycle in general.

A The cardiac cycle is the period from the end of one atrial contraction to the end of the next atrial contraction. Each heartbeat consists of a period of contraction, or systole, followed by a period of relaxation, or diastole. For example, if the heart beats 70 times per minute, each complete beat (systole and diastole) lasts 0.85 seconds. The atria and the ventricles do not contract simultaneously. The atria contract first, with atrial systole lasting 0.15 seconds. The ventricles then contract, with ventricular systole lasting 0.3 seconds. Diastole therefore lasts 0.4 seconds.

The cardiac cycle begins with atrial systole. The wave-like contraction of the atria is stimulated by the impulse of the sinoatrial or SA node. The contraction forces into the ventricles only 30 percent of the blood that will fill them. How the other 70 percent enters the ventricles will be explained shortly. During contraction of the two atria, the tricuspid and bicuspid valves are opened. There is a very brief pause before ventricular systole begins due to the delay in transmission of the cardiac impulse at the atrioventricular or AV node. The impulse is then transmitted to the AV bundle and bundle branches and then very rapidly to the Purkinje fibers, which stimulate the ventricles to contract as a unit. The contraction of the ventricular muscles causes a rapid increase in pressure in the ventricles. This increased ventricular pressure immediately closes the tricuspid and bicuspid valves, preventing backflow of the blood into the atria. It is important to realize that the valves work passively. There is no nervous stimulation that directly regulates their opening and closing; it is only the difference in pressure due to the relative amount of blood in the atria and ventricles (or ventricles and arteries) that controls this. As ventricular systole progresses, the ventricular pressure further increases (due to contraction). At this point, no blood is entering the ventricles, since the tri- and bicuspid valves are closed, and no blood is leaving, since the semilunar valves are closed. When the ventricular pressure becomes greater than the pressure in the arteries (the pulmonary artery and the aorta), the semilunar valves open, and blood is forced into these vessels. After the ventricles complete their contraction, ventricular diastole begins. As the ventricles relax, the pressure decreases. When the ventricular pressure is less than arterial pressure, the semilunar valves shut, preventing backflow. Since the pressure in the ventricles is still higher than in the atria, the tricuspid and bicuspid valves are still closed, and no blood enters or leaves the ventricles. But some blood is entering the now relaxed atria. During further relaxation of the ventricles, the ventricular pressure continues to decrease until it falls below the atrial pressure. At this point, the tricuspid and bicuspid valves open, allowing blood to rapidly flow into the ventricles. The atria do not contract to force this blood into the ventricles. It is a passive flow due to the fact that the atrial pressure is greater than the ventricular pressure. This flow allows for 70 percent of the ventricular filling before atrial systole. Thus, the major amount of ventricular filling occurs during diastole, not atrial systole, as one might expect.

11.4 Blood Vessels – Structure and Function

Arteries are vessels that conduct blood away from the heart. They branch into arterioles, vessels that are smaller and more numerous. Veins are vessels that transport blood to the heart. They form by the collection of venules, vessels that are smaller and more numerous. To supply any region of the body, the blood circulates through the following sequence of vessels: **arteries - arterioles - capillaries - venules - veins**.

Capillaries are microscopic vessels that are very numerous. Their function is exchange, meaning a two-way transport.

The **systemic circulation** contains this sequence of vessels. Originating with the aorta, the blood in this circuit contains blood high in oxygen and low in carbon dioxide. As blood circulates systemically, oxygen and nutrients leave the blood of the capillaries and enter body cells. Carbon dioxide and waste products leave cells and enter the blood. The systemic blood returns by veins to the right atrium.

The **pulmonary circulation** is a shorter route, beginning with the pulmonary trunk connected to the right ventricle. It contains blood low in oxygen and high in carbon dioxide. This situation is reversed at the capillaries in the lungs. This circuit ends where the pulmonary veins enter the left atrium. The blood now has more oxygen and less carbon dioxide. As it passes through the left side of the heart, it enters the aorta and becomes part of the systemic circulation.

The wall of a capillary consists of one layer of flat epithelial cells (simple squamous epithelium). This is suitable for their exchange role. The walls of all other vessels contain three layers.

Fibrous connective tissue composes the outer layer of an artery or arteriole, the **tunica externa**.

The middle layer, the **tunica media**, consists of smooth muscle with elastic fibers. Contraction of the muscle tissue produces the constriction of the vessel, called vasoconstriction. Relaxation of this tissue produces vasodilation, an increase in the diameter of the vessel.

The inner layer, the **tunica intima**, consists of simple squamous epithelium (endothelium). It provides a smooth surface for the passage of blood through the vessel.

If viewed by a transverse section, a vein or venule has the same three layers. However, the middle layer is proportionately thinner than in the arteries. Also, the inner layer has extensions called **valves**. Valves prevent the backflow of blood. Therefore, the blood continues to flow toward the heart.

Arteries and arterioles are **elastic** and **contractile**, due to the thickness of their middle layer. The blood pressure in systemic arteries is high, as they are near the left ventricle, which influences this pressure by contraction. The pressure in these arteries is also **pulsatile**, meaning it fluctuates due to the systole and diastole of the left ventricle during the cardiac cycle. When blood arrives in the arterioles, the pressure is lower and not pulsatile.

Blood pressure, which is the same in all large systemic arteries throughout the body, can be measured by two numbers expressed in millimeters of mercury (mmHg). The higher number is the **systolic** pressure, produced during the contraction (systole) of the left ventricle. When this chamber is relaxed (diastole) during the last half of the cardiac cycle, the pressure drops to a lower number, the **diastolic** pressure. If, for example, the blood pressure is 120/80, 120 is the systolic pressure, 80 is the diastolic pressure. The **pulse pressure** is the difference in these two numbers. In the previous case, it is 40 millimeters.

Veins and venules have the opposite properties of arteries. They are not as elastic or contractile, due to a thinner middle layer. The blood pressure in systemic veins is much lower (i.e., 10 to 30 mm), as they are near the end of the circulatory pathway that returns blood to the right side of the heart. The pressure is not pulsatile. Whereas a **pulse** (pulse pressure) can be felt in an artery (e.g., radial artery in the wrist), it cannot be found in a vein.

Blood circulates from arteries to veins due to a pressure difference, moving continuously from regions of higher pressure to regions of lower pressure. From arteries and arterioles, blood arrives at the capillaries.

When blood enters the systemic capillaries, the blood pressure is sufficient to force some plasma out into the intercellular spaces. Here it becomes **interstitial**. This fluid contains substances (e.g., oxygen) to supply body cells.

At the opposite end of the capillaries, the blood pressure has dropped significantly. It is less than the osmotic pressure that draws the fluid back into the capillaries. The osmotic pressure is due to the presence of plasma proteins in the blood. They make the blood hypertonic, causing it to draw fluid from the tissue spaces by osmosis; therefore, most of the tissue fluid returns to the capillaries at this end.

The tissue fluid entering the blood in the capillaries carries waste products from body cells. This blood enters the systemic venules and veins.

11.4.1 Circulation – Arteries and Veins

Arteries - All major arteries subdivide into smaller arteries that form arterioles. These arterioles deliver the blood to millions of capillaries that supply body regions.

The **aorta** is the largest artery. Beginning as the ascending aorta from the left ventricle, it forms an **arch**. Three major arteries distribute blood from the arch, delivering it to the head and arms. The **left subclavian** artery is lateral to the **left common carotid** artery. On the right side of the arch, the **brachiocephalic** (innominate) artery leaving the arch splits into the **right common carotid** and **right subclavian** arteries. The common carotid on each side subdivides into an external and internal carotid artery which supply the head and neck with blood.

The subclavian artery on each side supplies the arm by the following series of arteries: **axillary, brachial, radial, ulnar**. Blood flows through them in a distal direction. The subclavian becomes the axillary at the armpit. The axillary becomes the brachial as it parallels the humerus. In the forearm, blood enters the radial artery laterally and the ulnar artery medially.

Beyond the aortic arch, the aorta descends posterior to the heart. It continues to transport blood through the thorax and abdomen. Some arteries that branch from the **descending aorta** are:

Celiac - Supplies the stomach, liver, and spleen

Superior Mesenteric - Mainly supplies the small intestine

Renal - A pair of arteries supplies the kidneys

Inferior Mesenteric - Supplies most of the large intestine

At the level of the ilium of each hip bone, the aorta subdivides into two **common iliac** arteries. Each common iliac artery forms an **external** and **internal** artery. The internal iliac passes medially into the pelvic cavity, supplying the urinary and reproductive organs.

Each external iliac artery supplies the leg by the following series of arteries: **femoral, popliteal, anterior, posterior tibial**. The blood flows through them in a distal direction. The femoral artery begins in the upper three-fourths of the thigh. It has a branch, the **deep femoral artery**. The femoral becomes the popliteal in the posterior region of the knee. From the popliteal, blood flows into the two tibial arteries in the front and back of the shinbone.

Veins - Blood from the systemic capillaries collects into venules that transport the blood into larger and larger veins as it returns to the heart. The **superior** and **inferior vena cava** are the two thickest veins of the body, returning blood to the right atrium.

The head and arms are drained by four veins—two **internal jugular** veins that are larger than the external veins and medial, plus two **external jugular** veins that are smaller and lateral. Each internal jugular vein drains into a **brachiocephalic** (innominate) vein. These two veins form a V, merging to send blood into the superior vena cava. Each external jugular connects to a **subclavian** vein that drains the arm.

Distal to each subclavian vein, three major veins collect blood from each upper arm. The **cephalic** vein is lateral to the humerus. The **basilic** vein is medial. The **brachial** vein is posterior to the humerus. Near the proximal end of the humerus, the brachial and basilic veins form the **axillary** vein. The axillary vein sends blood to the subclavian vein. Laterally, the cephalic vein drains into the subclavian directly.

In the elbow region, some blood from the lateral forearm does not enter the cephalic vein but crosses over to the basilic through the **medial cubital** vein.

An **accessory cephalic** vein drains the lateral forearm, connecting to the cephalic vein at the elbow.

Two major venous routes drain blood from the leg. Laterally, the blood flows through this sequence of veins, moving in a proximal direction: **anterior and posterior tibial, popliteal, femoral, external iliac**. Medially, blood passes from the **dorsal venous arch** in the foot into the **great saphenous** vein, the longest vein of the body. The great saphenous vein connects to the femoral vein near the proximal end of the femur.

Each external iliac vein merges with an **internal iliac** vein, which is medial and drains the structures in the pelvic cavity. This merger forms the **common iliac** vein on each side. The two common iliac veins form the inferior vena cava. As the second longest vein, it transports blood through the abdomen and thorax, returning it to the right atrium.

Hepatic Portal System - Many organs in the abdominal cavity are drained by veins that deliver blood to the liver before it is released into the inferior vena cava for return to the heart. At the liver, this blood passes through another series of capillaries. This hepatic portal circulation ranges from the capillaries of the following organs to the capillaries of the liver: pancreas, gallbladder, spleen, stomach, small intestine, and large intestine.

The liver controls the concentration of glucose, toxins, and other substances in the blood passing through it. After these adjustments are made, the capillaries in the liver collect into larger vessels, forming the hepatic vein. It transports blood into the inferior vena cava.

11.5 Lymphatic System

The lymphatic circulation is sometimes considered a separate system from the rest of the circulatory system. It begins with **lymph capillaries**, microscopic vessels that take up a product of the tissue fluid not recaptured by the nearby systemic capillaries. This fluid is called **lymph**. It contains more protein than normal tissue fluid.

The lymph capillaries collect into larger and larger vessels, the lymphatics. These lymphatics parallel the systemic venules and veins in body regions, but contain more valves. The final two collecting vessels are the **thoracic duct** and **right lymphatic duct**. The right lymphatic duct drains the right arm and right halves of the head and thorax. The thoracic duct drains the remainder of the body. Both of these vessels add lymph to the systemic blood in veins near the heart.

Lymph nodes are found at certain sites of the lymphatic circulation. The major lymph nodes are the cervical, axillary, cubital, and inguinal. The nodes contain phagocytic cells that filter the blood and fight infection. In addition, some lymphocytes are produced in the lymph nodes.

Lymph capillaries in the wall of the small intestine absorb fatty acids from the diet.

Problem Solving Example:

Q The lymphatic system in humans constitutes an extensive network of thin vessels resembling veins. What are the functions of the lymphatic system?

A The lymphatic system is not part of the circulatory system per se, but constitutes a one-way route from interstitial fluid to the blood. The lymphatic system in humans constitutes an extensive network of thin-walled vessels resembling the veins. These vessels ultimately drain into veins in the lower neck. One of the functions of the lymphatic system is to transfer excess interstitial fluid back to the blood. There is a net movement of plasma out of the capillaries and into the tissues; the lymphatics restore the blood volume by returning this fluid that has filtered out. In addition, the lymphatic system serves to return proteins to the blood. Since the capillaries have a slight permeability to plasma proteins, and since the concentration of protein in the blood plasma is greater than that in the interstitial fluid, there is a small but steady loss of protein from the blood into the interstitial fluid. This protein returns to the blood via the lymphatics. Should there be a malfunction in the lymphatic system, the interstitial fluid protein concentration would increase to that of the plasma. This eliminates the protein concentration difference between the plasma and the interstitial fluid, thus eliminating the plasma colloid osmotic pressure. Only blood pressure and interstitial fluid pressure remain, and permit the net movement of fluid out of the capillary into the interstitial space (edema).

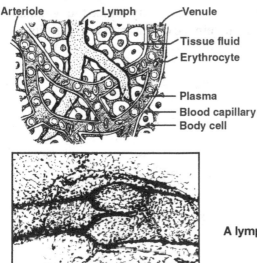

Arteriole Lymph Venule

Tissue fluid

Erythrocyte

Plasma

Blood capillary

Body cell

Diagram of the relation of blood and lymph capillaries to tissue cells. Note that blood capillaries are connected at both ends, whereas lymph capillaries, outlined in black, are "dead-end streets" and contain no erythrocytes. The arrows indicate direction of flow.

A lymph vessel valve

Another function of the lymphatic system is to provide the pathway by which fat and other substances absorbed from the gut reach the blood. It is also believed that certain high molecular weight hormones reach the blood via the lymphatics.

In addition to its function in transport, the lymphatic system plays a critical role in the body's defense mechanism against disease. The lymph nodes, which are found at the junctions of lymph vessels, act as filters and are sites of formation of certain types of white blood cells. Lymph, the fluid in the lymph capillaries, flows slowly through the nodes, where invading bacteria are phagocytosed by the cells of the lymph node. Indigestible particles such as dust and soot, which the phagocytic cells cannot destroy, are stored in the nodes. Since the nodes are particularly active during an infection, they often become swollen and sore, as the lymph nodes at the base of the jaw are apt to become during a throat infection.

It should be noted that since the lymphatic system is not connected to the arterial portion of the blood circulatory system, lymph is not moved by the hydrostatic pressure developed by the heart. Lymph flow, like that in the veins, depends primarily upon forces external to the vessels. These forces include the contractile action of the skeletal muscle (through which the lymphatics flow) and the effects of respiration on the pressures in the chest cavity. Since the lymphatics have valves similar to those in veins, external pressure permits only unidirectional flow.

Quiz: The Circulatory System

1. Highest pressure of circulating blood is found in a(n)

   (A) arteriole.   (D) vein.

   (B) artery.   (E) venule.

   (C) capillary.

2. A person receives the results of a hematocrit during a series of blood tests. A hematocrit is the

   (A) abundance of white blood cells in the blood.

   (B) concentration of sugar in the blood.

   (C) level of circulating antibodies.

   (D) percentage of blood cellular material by volume.

   (E) typing of the blood by the ABO scheme.

3. A universal recipient is a person who has which type of blood?

   (A) A+   (D) O+

   (B) AB+   (E) O–

   (C) AB–

4. A person's blood pressure is taken, revealing a diastolic pressure of 90 mmHg. The pulse pressure is 30 mmHg. The systolic pressure is

   (A) 30 mmHg.

   (B) 60 mmHg.

   (C) 90 mmHg.

(D) 120 mmHg.

(E) 270 mmHg.

5. The pumping chambers of the heart are called the

    (A) atria.

    (B) ventricles.

    (C) pacemakers.

    (D) cardiac muscles.

    (E) vena cava.

6. Which statement about blood circulation in the heart is correct?

    (A) The right ventricle pumps blood to the systemic circulation.

    (B) Blood enters the right atrium from the inferior vena cava.

    (C) Blood enters the left atrium from the superior vena cava.

    (D) Blood enters the right atrium from the pulmonary arteries.

    (E) Blood enters the left atrium directly from the right ventricle.

7. Lymph is moved by

    (A) diffusion.

    (B) pressure from the heart.

    (C) a special lymph pump.

    (D) differing osmotic pressure in the capillaries.

    (E) active transport.

8. If the blood pressure of a human is 111/80,

    (A) the systolic pressure is 80.

    (B) the diastolic pressure is 80.

    (C) the pulse rate is 80 beats per minute.

    (D) the blood pressure during contraction of the heart is 80.

    (E) the right atrium moved 110 ml of blood per beat, and the left atrium moved 80 ml of blood per beat.

9. Which of the following correctly shows the path of blood in the blood vessels?

    (A) Arterioles - capillaries - arteries - veins - venules

    (B) Arteries - arterioles - capillaries - venules - veins

    (C) Capillaries - arterioles - arteries - veins - venules

    (D) Venules - capillaries - veins - arteries - venules

    (E) Veins - venules - arterioles - capillaries - arteries

10. Memory cells produced by B-lymphocytes help the organism to respond more quickly to an infection the second time because they

    (A) start a cell-mediated response.

    (B) have created their own antigens from the first exposure to the infection.

    (C) rapidly clone antibodies picked up during the first exposure to the infection.

    (D) directly attack the invaders instead of producing antibodies.

    (E) are not specific to a particular antigen.

ANSWER KEY

1.	(B)		6.	(B)
2.	(D)		7.	(D)
3.	(B)		8.	(B)
4.	(D)		9.	(B)
5.	(B)		10.	(C)

CHAPTER 12

The Respiratory System

12.1 Respiration

Respiration is a process that involves the distribution and use of gases, oxygen, and carbon dioxide by the body. It occurs at several different levels:

1. **Breathing** - The inhalation and exhalation of air

2. **External respiration** - The exchange of gases between the lungs and the blood of the pulmonary capillaries

3. **Internal respiration** - The exchange of gases between the blood of the systemic capillaries and cells

Inhaled and exhaled air passes through a series of chambers during inhalation and exhalation. These chambers are continuous and are structures of the respiratory tract. Inhaled air passes through the chambers of this tract in the following order:

nose - pharynx - larynx - trachea - primary bronchus -

secondary bronchus - bronchioles - alveolar ducts - alveoli - lungs

Problem Solving Example:

Q Differentiate between breathing and respiration.

A Respiration has two distinct meanings. It refers to the oxidative degradation of nutrients such as glucose through metabolic reactions within the cell, resulting in the production of carbon dioxide, water, and energy. Respiration also refers to the exchange of gases between the cells of an organism and the external environment. Many different methods for exchange are used by different organisms. In humans, respiration can be categorized by three phases: ventilation (breathing), external respiration, and internal respiration.

Breathing may be defined as the mechanical process of taking air into the lungs (inhalation) and expelling it (exhalation). It does not include the exchange of gases between the bloodstream and the alveoli. Breathing must occur in order for respiration to occur; that is, air must be brought to the alveolar cells before exchange can be effective. One distinction that can be made between respiration and breathing is that the former ultimately results in energy production in the cells. Breathing, on the other hand, is solely an energy consuming process because of the muscular activity required to move the diaphragm.

12.1.1 Anatomy – Respiratory Tract

Nose - The external nose projects from the face. The larger internal nose is superior to the oral cavity, separated from it by the hard palate. Several bones of the skull (e.g., ethmoid) are the boundaries of the internal nose.

Inhaled air passes through a pair of **external nares** (nostrils) of the external nose. The mucous membranes lining the internal nose moisten and filter the air. The plentiful blood supply in these membranes also warms the air. Olfactory receptors in the roof of the internal nose detect different chemicals in the air, initiating the sense of olfaction (smell).

Pharynx - Inhaled air passes through a pair of internal nares in the posterior portion of the internal nose. From these openings air enters the pharynx (throat). This muscular tube, about five inches in length, is lined with mucous membranes.

Vertically, the throat consists of three regions: the **nasopharynx**, **oropharynx**, and **laryngopharynx**. The nasopharynx extends from the internal nares to the level of the soft palate of the oral cavity. The oropharynx extends from this palate to the hyoid bone. The laryngo-pharynx is the remaining inferior portion of the throat.

The throat has several pairs of tonsils that protect the body from invading bacteria. The pharyngeal tonsils (adenoids), for example, are in the posterior wall of the nasopharynx.

Larynx - The larynx (voicebox) consists of nine pieces of carti-lage. The three largest pieces are the **epiglottis, thyroid cartilage**, and **cricoid cartilage**.

The epiglottis is the superior, leaf-like part of the larynx. It is at-tached to the larynx posteriorly, capable of covering its opening at the top, the **glottis**. It normally covers this opening when food is swallowed. The thyroid cartilage (Adam's apple) is the large, triangular piece. The cricoid cartilage is the most inferior piece, attaching the larynx to the first ring of the trachea.

Folds of the mucous membranes lining the inside of the larynx, the **vocal cords**, extend across the interior of this structure. Skeletal muscles cause them to vibrate at different frequencies, determining the pitch of voice production.

Trachea - The trachea (windpipe) is a tube about five inches long and one inch in diameter. Its wall of smooth muscle is reinforced with rings of C-shaped cartilage. The open end of the C's is directed toward the esophagus of the digestive tract, which is posterior to the trachea. The trachea is lined with mucous membranes.

Primary Bronchus - The base of the trachea subdivides into a left and right primary (main) bronchus. This arrangement resembles an inverted Y, with each bronchus entering one of the lungs. Each lung is an elastic, bag-like structure that houses the remainder of the respiratory tract. The left lung is smaller than the right lung.

Secondary Bronchus - Each primary bronchus subdivides into secondary bronchi. There are three secondary bronchi in the right lung, one serving each lobe of the lung (three lobes). There are two secondary bronchi in the left lung, one serving each lobe of this lung (two lobes).

Bronchioles - The tract continues to subdivide into smaller, more numerous passageways in the lung. This pattern resembles an inverted tree. Bronchioles are very small tubes, lacking the cartilage rings found in the bronchi.

Alveolar Ducts and Alveoli - Most of the interior of the lungs is filled with microscopic air sacs called alveoli (singular, alveolus). The alveoli exist as clusters. Each one in a group receives inhaled air from an alveolar duct. The pair of lungs has an estimated 300 million alveoli. The alveoli are close to the capillaries of the pulmonary circulation. The thin walls of the alveoli consist of one layer of cells, simple squamous epithelium.

Lungs - Each lung has a broad, inferior base that rests on the diaphragm. Its apex is the cone-shaped, superior portion, projecting about one inch above the clavicle. Most of the surfaces of the lung are costal, facing and contacting the ribs.

Each lung resides within an **intrapleural cavity**. This is a sealed off space within two layers of serous membranes. The **parietal pleura** lines the inside surface of the chest wall. The **pulmonary pleura** adheres to the lung.

The pressure in the intrapleural cavity is normally negative, meaning that it is below atmospheric pressure. At standard conditions of sea level, atmospheric pressure is 760 mmHg when measured by a barometer. If, for example, the intrapleural pressure is 757 mmHg, it is three units below this (−3 compared to a standard of 0).

Problem Solving Example:

Identify the parts of the human respiratory system. How is each adapted for its particular function?

The respiratory system in humans and other air-breathing vertebrates includes the lungs and the tubes by which air reaches them. Normally, air enters the human respiratory system by way of the external nares or nostrils, but it may also enter by way of the mouth. The nostrils, which contain small hairs to filter incoming air, lead into the nasal cavities, which are separated from the mouth below by the palate. The nasal cavities contain the sense organs of smell, and are lined with mucus-secreting epithelium, which moistens the incoming air. Air passes from the nasal cavities via the internal nares into the pharynx, then through the glottis and into the larynx. The larynx is often called the Adam's apple, and is more prominent in men than women. Stretched across the larynx are the vocal cords. The opening to the larynx, called the glottis, is always open except in swallowing, when a flap-like structure (the epiglottis) covers it. Leading from the larynx to the chest region is a long cylindrical tube called the trachea, or windpipe. In a dissection, the trachea can be distinguished from the esophagus by its cartilaginous C-shaped rings, which serve to hold the tracheal tube open. In the middle of the chest, the trachea bifurcates into bronchi, which lead to the lungs. In the lungs, each bronchus branches, forming smaller and smaller tubes called bronchioles. The smaller bronchioles terminate in clusters of cup-shaped cavities, the air sacs. In the walls of the smaller bronchioles and the air sacs are the alveoli, which are moist structures supplied with a rich network of capillaries. Molecules of oxygen and carbon dioxide diffuse readily through the thin, moist walls of the alveoli. The total alveolar surface area across which gases may diffuse has been estimated to be greater than 100 square meters.

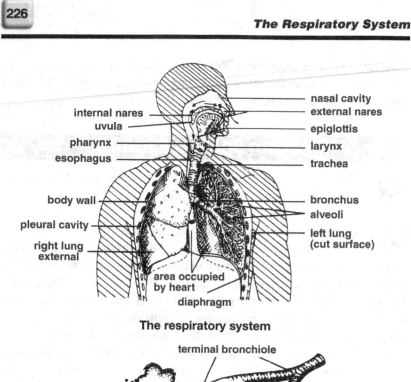

internal nares
uvula
pharynx
esophagus

nasal cavity
external nares
epiglottis
larynx
trachea

body wall
pleural cavity
right lung
external

bronchus
alveoli
left lung
(cut surface)

area occupied
by heart
diaphragm

The respiratory system

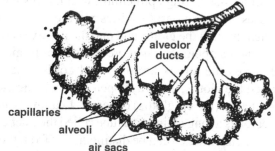

terminal bronchiole

alveolor
ducts

capillaries
alveoli
air sacs

Diagram of a small portion of the lung, highly magnified, showing the air sacs at the end of the alveolar ducts, the alveoli in the walls of the air sacs, and the proximity of the alveoli and the pulmonary capillaries containing red blood cells

Each lung, as well as the cavity of the chest in which the lung rests, is covered by a thin sheet of smooth epithelium, the pleura. The pleura is kept moist, enabling the lungs to move without much friction during breathing. The pleura actually consists of two layers of membranes that are continuous with each other at the point at which the bronchus enters the lung, called the hilus (roof). Thus, the pleura is more correctly a sac than a single sheet covering the lungs.

The chest cavity is closed and has no communication with the outside. It is bounded by the chest wall, which contains the ribs on its top, sides and back, and the sternum anteriorly. The bottom of the chest wall is covered by a strong, dome-shaped sheet of skeletal muscle, the diaphragm. The diaphragm separates the chest region (thorax) from the abdominal region, and plays a crucial role in breathing by contracting and relaxing, changing the intrathoracic pressure.

12.2 Breathing – Physiology

Breathing is a cycle involving the alternation of two processes, inhalation and exhalation. Each process unfolds through a series of steps, beginning with a pressure in the lungs of 0 (760 mm).

Inhalation - The inflow of air results from a series of volume and pressure changes. The process of inhalation includes the following steps:

1. The **respiratory center** in the medulla sends a signal to the **diaphragm** and **intercostal muscles**. This signal causes these skeletal muscles to contract.

2. When relaxed, the diaphragm is elevated. As it contracts, it flattens, increasing the size of the intrapleural cavity vertically. The intercostal muscles also contract, elevating the ribs. This increases the size of the intrapleural cavity transversely.

3. As the size of the intrapleural cavity increases, the pressure inside of it decreases. This inverse relationship between volume and pressure is stated by **Boyle's law**. With a normal, quiet inhalation (tidal volume), the pressure in the cavity drops from –3 to –6.

4. The lungs are drawn into the region of lower pressure in the intrapleural cavity surrounding them. As their volume increases, the pressure inside them decreases. With a normal inhalation, the pressure in the lungs drops from 0 to –3.

5. The pressure in the lungs, particularly the alveoli, drops below atmospheric pressure. The pressure in the lungs is now −3 compared to 0 (760 mm) in the atmosphere.

6. Air is drawn from the region of higher pressure (atmosphere, 0) to the region of lower pressure (lungs, −3). As a result, air rushes into the lungs, producing an inhalation.

Problem Solving Example:

 Explain the physical changes that take place during inhalation.

 Just before inhalation, at the conclusion of the previous exhalation, the respiratory muscles are relaxed, and no air is flowing into or out of the lungs. Inhalation is initiated by the contraction of the dome-shaped diaphragm and the intercostal muscles. When the diaphragm contracts, it moves downward into the abdomen. Simultaneously, the intercostal muscles on the ribs contract, leading to

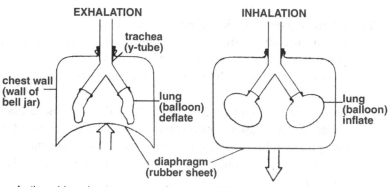

EXHALATION   INHALATION

trachea (y-tube)

chest wall (wall of bell jar)

lung (balloon) deflate

lung (balloon) inflate

diaphragm (rubber sheet)

As the rubber sheet moves up, the volume in a bell jar decreases with a corresponding increase in pressure within the jar. This causes air to rush out of the Y-tube, resulting in the collapse of the balloon.

When the rubber sheet moves down, the volume increases with a corresponding decrease in pressure. Thus, the balloons inflate.

Model of how the diaphragm works

an upward and outward movement of the ribs. As a result of these two physical changes the volume of the chest cavity increases and hence the pressure within the chest decreases. Then, the atmospheric pressure, which is now greater than the intrathoracic pressure, forces air to enter the lungs, and causes them to inflate or expand. During exhalation, the intercostal muscles relax, and the ribs move downward and inward. At the same time, the diaphragm relaxes and resumes its original dome shape. Consequently the thoracic volume returns to its pre-inhalation state, and the pressure within the chest increases. This increase in pressure, together with the elastic recoil of the lungs, forces air out of the lungs, causing them to deflate. The role of the diaphragm in breathing is demonstrated by the figure on the previous page.

Exhalation - The outflow of air results from a series of volume and pressure changes that reverse the situation that produced an inhalation. The process of exhalation includes the following steps:

1. The diaphragm relaxes, returning to an elevated position. The intercostal muscles relax, causing the ribs to drop.

2. The relaxation of these skeletal muscles decreases the size of the intrapleural cavity.

3. As the size of the cavity decreases, the pressure in the cavity increases. With a normal exhalation, this increase is from about –6 to –3.

4. The lungs are compressed somewhat by the decrease in the volume of the intrapleural cavity around them. As their volume decreases, the pressure in them increases.

5. The pressure in the lungs is also increased by the recoil of the elastic tissue in their walls. This recoil causes the pressure in the lungs to become temporarily positive (i.e., +3 or +4).

6. Air is forced from the region of higher pressure (lungs, +3) to the region of lower pressure (atmosphere, 0). As a result, air moves out of the lungs, producing an exhalation.

When the positive pressure in the lungs drops back to 0, the cycle is completed and can begin again.

The volume of air that is inhaled or exhaled can vary depending on the metabolic needs of the body. Air volumes, measured through **spirometry** in the laboratory, include:

Tidal volume (TV) - Volume of air normally inhaled or exhaled by quiet breathing. An average tidal volume is 500 ml.

Expiratory reserve volume (ERV) - This is the amount of air that can be exhaled in addition to the tidal volume. It can be as much as 1,000 ml.

Inspiratory reserve volume (IRV) - This is the amount of air that can be inhaled in addition to the tidal volume. In some individuals this can be as high as 3,000 ml.

Vital capacity (VC) - This is the total lung capacity. It is the sum of the tidal volume plus the two reserves:

$$VC = TV + IRV + ERV$$

Residual volume - This is a remaining volume of air in the lungs that cannot be forcibly expired. It can range from 800 to 1,000 ml.

The rate and depth (volume) of breathing changes to meet the changing requirements of body metabolism. The total volume of air inhaled or exhaled per minute can be computed by multiplying rate and depth. For example:

$$12 \text{ cycles/min} \times 500 \text{ ml} = 6,000 \text{ ml}$$

The respiratory center in the medulla will increase rate and depth if the level of carbon dioxide and hydrogen ions (acidity) increases in the arterial blood. This increase eliminates these waste products. Also, as the body breathes faster and deeper, more needed oxygen is acquired.

Problem Solving Example:

 What is meant by the "vital capacity" of a person? In what conditions is it increased or decreased?

During a single normal breath, the volume of air entering or leaving the lungs is called the tidal volume. Under conditions of rest, this volume is approximately 500 ml on average. The volume of air that can be inspired over and above the resting tidal volume is called the inspiratory reserve volume, and amounts to about 3,000 ml of air. Similarly, the volume of air that can be expired below the resting tidal volume is called the expiratory reserve volume, and amounts to approximately 1,000 ml of air. Even after forced maximum expiration, some air (about 1,000 ml) still remains in the lungs, and is termed the residual volume. The vital capacity is the sum of the tidal volume and the inspiratory and expiratory reserve volumes. The vital capacity then represents the maximum amount of air that can be moved in and out during a single breath. The average vital capacity varies with gender, being 4.5 liters for the young adult male and about 3.2 liters for the young adult female. During heavy work or exercise, a person uses part of both the inspiratory and expiratory reserves, but rarely uses more

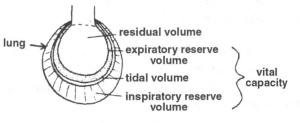

Lung volumes

than 50 percent of his or her total vital capacity. This is because deeper breaths than this would require exhaustive activities of the inspiratory and expiratory muscles. Vital capacity is higher in an individual who is tall and thin than in one who is obese. A well-developed athlete may have a vital capacity up to 55 percent above average. In some diseases of the heart and lungs, the vital capacity may be reduced considerably.

12.3 External Respiration

Blood transported from the right side of the heart has a low concentration of oxygen and a high concentration of carbon dioxide. As this blood arrives in the capillaries of the pulmonary circulation, these situations are reversed by the exchange processes of external respiration. The events of these processes are:

1. Oxygen diffuses from the alveoli into the blood.

2. Carbon dioxide diffuses from the blood into the alveoli.

The concentrations of gases are expressed by **partial pressures**. Each gas in a mixture of gases contributes its part to the entire gas pressure. For example, in the atmosphere, the partial pressure of oxygen is about 152 mmHg. This is because oxygen comprises about 20 percent of the total air pressure ($0.2 \times 760 = 152$).

The partial pressure of oxygen in the alveoli is often around 100. In the blood of the pulmonary capillaries, it is much lower (i.e., 35). Therefore, oxygen diffuses from the alveoli into the blood, raising the pressure in the blood to about 100.

The partial pressure of carbon dioxide in the alveoli is low, perhaps around 40. In the blood of the pulmonary capillaries, it is higher, at about 48. Therefore, carbon dioxide diffuses from the blood into the alveoli, dropping the pressure in the blood to about 40.

Diffusion is a transport process that tends toward an equilibrium. Therefore, all blood returning to the left side of the heart has partial pressures that have changed to about:

oxygen: 100 (up from 35)
carbon dioxide: 40 (down from 48)

Each pressure represents the level in the alveolus. The blood has equilibrated with concentrations close to these levels.

12.4 Internal Respiration

The blood returns to the left side of the heart after external respiration. It is pumped through the aorta from the left ventricle, reaching tissue cells by the systemic circulation. In the systemic capillaries, the processes of internal respiration occur. These processes are:

1. Oxygen diffuses from the blood into the tissue cells.

2. Carbon dioxide diffuses from the tissue cells into the blood.

Oxygen is used as a reactant by cellular respiration. Cellular respiration also produces carbon dioxide, which is a waste product that must be eliminated from tissue cells.

The partial pressure of oxygen in the blood of the systemic capillaries is often about 100. In the tissue cells, it is about 40. Therefore, oxygen diffuses into the cells.

The partial pressure of carbon dioxide in the blood of the systemic capillaries is about 40. In the tissue cells it can be 48. Therefore, carbon dioxide diffuses into the blood.

By equilibration through diffusion, the partial pressures for the blood returning to the right side of the heart are about:

oxygen: 35 (down from 100)
carbon dioxide: 48 (up from 40)

For each amount of blood returning to the lungs, these values for partial pressures are changed again through the processes of external respiration. As a summary, one example of these changes is:

oxygen: 35 to 100 as the blood acquires this gas from the lungs by external respiration; 100 to 35 as the blood loses some of this gas to cells by internal respiration

carbon dioxide: 48 to 40 as the cells lose some of this gas by external respiration; 40 to 48 as the blood acquires this gas from the cells by internal respiration

Problem Solving Example:

Q Differentiate between external and internal respiration.

A Gas exchange between the body cells and the environment (indirect respiration) may be categorized into two phases: an external and an internal phase. External respiration is the exchange of gases by diffusion that occurs between the lungs and the bloodstream. Oxygen passes from the lungs to the blood and carbon dioxide passes from the blood to the lungs. Internal respiration takes place throughout the body. In the latter, there is an exchange of gases between the blood and other tissues of the body, with oxygen passing from the blood to the tissue cells and carbon dioxide passing from the cells to the blood. This phase, along with the external phase, relies on the movement of gases from a region of higher concentration to one of lower concentration.

Quiz: The Respiratory System

1. Which law explains the inhalation and exhalation of air in terms of pressure changes?

    (A) Archimedes' law

    (B) Aristotle's law

    (C) Boyle's law

    (D) Dalton's law

    (E) Mendel's law

2. A respiratory system does not necessarily need

    (A) an exchange surface with an adequate area.

    (B) a means to transport gases to internal areas.

    (C) a means of protecting exchange surfaces.

    (D) moist gas exchange surfaces.

    (E) a location deep inside an organism.

3. The volume of air entering or leaving the lungs during a single normal breath is called the

    (A) vital capacity.

    (B) tidal volume.

    (C) breathing capacity.

    (D) residual volume.

    (E) inspiratory or expiratory reserve volume.

4. The diffusion of CO_2 from the tissue spaces to the blood is called

   (A) external respiration.

   (B) ventilation.

   (C) internal respiration.

   (D) inspiratory capacity.

   (E) respiratory capacity.

5. Another name for the throat is the

   (A) esophagus.

   (B) larynx.

   (C) nasal cavity.

   (D) pharynx.

   (E) trachea.

6. Exhaled air flows through the tract passages by the sequence

   (A) alveolus - bronchus - trachea - bronchiole - larynx.

   (B) alveolus - bronchiole - bronchus - trachea - larynx.

   (C) bronchiole - alveolus - trachea - larynx - bronchus.

   (D) bronchiole - trachea - larynx - bronchus - alveolus.

   (E) larynx - trachea - bronchus - bronchiole - alveolus.

7. Which one of the following structures of the respiratory tract is made up of smooth muscle reinforced with rings of C-shaped cartilage?

   (A) Larynx   (D) Trachea

   (B) Pharynx   (E) Bronchioles

   (C) Vocal cords

8. Vital capacity is equal to which one of the following?

    (A) Tidal volume + residual volume

    (B) Tidal volume + inspiratory reserve volume

    (C) Tidal volume + expiratory reserve volume

    (D) Tidal volume + inspiratory reserve volume + expiratory reserve volume

    (E) Tidal volume + inspiratory reserve volume − expiratory reserve volume

9. What is the total volume of air inhaled per minute if a person has a tidal volume of 600 ml and breathes at a rate of 11 cycles per minute?

    (A) 55 ml

    (B) 66 ml

    (C) 250 ml

    (D) 1,000 ml

    (E) 6,600 ml

10. The respiratory center of the medulla will increase the rate and depth of breathing if, in the arterial blood, the level of

    (A) CO_2 increases.

    (B) CO_2 decreases.

    (C) hydrogen ions increase.

    (D) Both (A) and (C).

    (E) Both (B) and (C).

ANSWER KEY

1.	(C)	6.	(B)
2.	(E)	7.	(D)
3.	(B)	8.	(D)
4.	(C)	9.	(E)
5.	(D)	10.	(D)

CHAPTER 13

The Digestive System

13.1 Digestion

Most molecules in the human diet are too large to be used in metabolism. Starch, as one example, is a complex carbohydrate. This polysaccharide is too large to be absorbed into the bloodstream and transported by circulation.

The digestive system prepares food molecules for use in the body. It accomplishes this through physical digestion and chemical digestion.

13.1.1 Physical Digestion

Part of the digestion of food involves a physical change. Masses of food are broken into smaller particles without altering the chemical structure of the molecules. Physical digestion begins in the oral cavity with mastication (chewing). Another example occurs in the small intestine, where the secretion of bile emulsifies fat globules, subdividing them into smaller droplets.

13.1.2 Chemical Digestion

Chemical digestion occurs when the chemical makeup of dietary molecules is changed. Starch is changed into the disaccharide maltose in the oral cavity. Later, in the small intestine, all disaccharides are converted into monosaccharides such as glucose. Throughout the digestive tract, organic catalysts, called enzymes, accelerate these chemical changes. In the oral cavity, for example, the enzyme amylase increases the rate by which starch is converted into the sugar maltose.

13.2 Anatomy – Digestive Tract and Accessory Structures

Most of the anatomy of the digestive system consists of a series of continuous chambers found on the ventral side of the body. They belong to a digestive tract that is more than 30 feet in length. Food passes through the following series of chambers of this tract: **oral cavity - pharynx - esophagus - stomach - small intestine - large intestine - rectum**.

Several accessory structures also belong to the digestive system. These structures are either found in chambers, such as the **salivary glands** and **teeth**, or are structures that connect to the tract. The **liver**, **gallbladder**, and **pancreas** all connect by ducts to the duodenum, the first segment of the small intestine.

Oral Cavity - The oral cavity contains 32 permanent (secondary) teeth. There are four tooth types based on their unique shape and size. The anterior **incisors** have sharp edges for cutting. The **canine** teeth have some ability to tear food. The **premolars** and **molars** have broad, flat crowns for crushing and grinding food. In any one of the four quadrants (quarters) of the mouth, there are eight teeth: two incisors (central and lateral), one canine (lateral and posterior to the lateral incisor), two premolars (posterior to the canine), and three molars (posterior to the premolars). The third molar (most posterior) is the wisdom tooth.

A tooth has three layers: the outer **enamel**, the **dentin** (middle layer), and inner **pulp**. The white enamel is the hardest substance in the body. The pulp contains the blood vessels and nerves.

The **crown** is the portion of the tooth, covered with enamel, above the line of the gingiva (gum). The **neck** is the constricted portion normally covered by the gum. The **root** is the part anchoring the tooth in the cancellous bone of either the maxilla or the mandible.

Several pairs of **salivary glands** secrete saliva through ducts into the oral cavity. The saliva contains amylase and moistens the food. Each **parotid gland** is embedded in the cheek, anterior and somewhat inferior to the ear. Each **submandibular gland** is near the posterior corner of the mandible. Each **sublingual gland** is under the mucous membrane lining the bottom of the oral cavity.

Skeletal muscles in the **tongue** contract to manipulate the food into a ball, or bolus, for swallowing. The surface of the tongue also contains the receptors for the sense of taste.

Pharynx - Food passes into the oropharynx through an opening from the oral cavity, the fauces.

Esophagus - The esophagus is a 10-inch muscular tube that accepts food from the pharynx. Peristalsis, rhythmic contractions of the tract wall, squeezes food along to the stomach.

Stomach - The **fundus** is the superior cap of the stomach. The **body** is the thick main portion. The **pylorus** is the constricted portion connected to the small intestine. The **cardiac sphincter** is a circular arrangement of smooth muscle fibers where the esophagus meets the stomach. The **pyloric sphincter** at the other end of the stomach has a similar makeup. These sphincters are controlled by reflexes to contract at certain times, preventing the backflow of food.

The stomach is a reservoir storing food, passing it on in small increments to the small intestine. The chemical digestion of proteins begins in this chamber. The enzyme pepsin, working in an acid environment (pH of 1 to 3), speeds up this digestion. HCl secreted into the stomach accounts for this acidity. Peristaltic action of the smooth muscle in the stomach wall contributes to physical digestion.

The stomach has four layers, which are also found in the next several chambers of the digestive tract. From the inside they are the **mucosa** (mucous membrane), **submucosa** (containing blood vessels), **muscularis** (smooth muscle), and **serosa**.

Small Intestine - The small intestine consists of three regions. The **duodenum** is the first 10 to 12 inches. This C-shaped region is followed by the **jejunum** (8 feet). The last 12 feet is the **ileum**. The ileum is separated from the large intestine by the **ileocecal valve**.

The mucosa of the small intestine has **villi** (singular, villus), finger-like projections that greatly increase the surface area of this lining. The small intestine is the main site of **absorption**, the passage of nutrient molecules from the digestive tract into the bloodstream. The chemical digestion of carbohydrates and proteins is completed here. The chemical digestion of lipids is started and completed here.

The stomach and small intestine are connected to **mesenteries**, which are sheet-like folds of serous membranes. Mesenteries are a continuation of the serous lining of the abdominal cavity, the **peritoneum**. They store fat and also contain blood vessels and nerves that supply the digestive tract.

Several accessory structures secrete substances into the duodenum. The **pancreas** ranges from the C-shaped recess of the duodenum to along the bottom of the stomach. It secretes many enzymes, through a **pancreatic duct**, into the duodenum. It also secretes bicarbonate ions into this chamber. These ions buffer the acidic **chyme**, a mixture of partially digested food passing into the small intestine from the stomach. The buffering action neutralizes this acidity, making the small intestine slightly basic (pH of 8 to 9).

The **liver** consists of two lobes. The larger right lobe is across from the stomach. The liver has many metabolic functions, such as converting glucose into stored glycogen and detoxifying poisons. It also manufactures bile, a substance stored in the **gallbladder**. This bulb-like structure is under the right lobe of the liver. Bile, when secreted into the small intestine, emulsifies fats globules.

The gallbladder is drained by the **cystic duct**. The liver is drained by the **hepatic duct**. These two ducts merge to form the **common bile duct**, which connects to the duodenum.

Large Intestine - The large intestine, or colon, is five to eight feet long. Its regions are the:

Cecum - This is a pouch-like region where the ileum attaches. A thin appendix extends from it.

Ascending Colon - This rises vertically in the abdomen from the crest of the ilium on the right. It contacts the liver.

Transverse Colon - It meets the ascending colon at the hepatic flexure (bend). The transverse colon ranges across the liver and stomach, contacting the spleen on the left.

Descending Colon - It meets the transverse colon at the splenic flexure. This region of the large intestine extends from the spleen to the left iliac crest.

Sigmoid Colon - It is S-shaped, entering the pelvic cavity from the left iliac crest and ending medially.

The large intestine is the site of **reabsorption**. By this process most of the fluids from secretions added internally to the tract (e.g., saliva, gastric juice from the stomach) are reclaimed into the bloodstream. Whatever is not reabsorbed is **eliminated** from the body. The remaining feces, solid waste, consists of some fluid, undigested food molecules, dead cells, and bacteria that normally inhabit this lower portion of the tract. This mass passes through the rectum when eliminated.

Rectum - The rectum is the last seven to eight inches of the tract. Solid wastes pass through it and leave through the **anus**, the opening at the end of the tract.

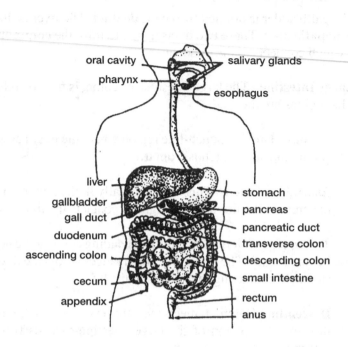

oral cavity

pharynx

salivary glands

esophagus

liver

gallbladder

gall duct

duodenum

ascending colon

cecum

appendix

stomach

pancreas

pancreatic duct

transverse colon

descending colon

small intestine

rectum

anus

The digestive system

13.3 Physiology of the Digestive System

Food is digested through physical and chemical changes. Hydrolysis is chemical digestion. By the insertion of a water molecule, a covalent bond can be broken, and larger molecules are reduced to smaller subunits. This occurs in three chambers of the tract. They are the oral cavity, stomach, and small intestine.

13.3.1 Hydrolysis

Oral Cavity - Salivary amylase accelerates the hydrolysis of starch into maltose. This change only begins here. Amylase is an enzyme that functions best at the pH of 7 in this cavity. The hydrolysis of proteins and lipids does not begin yet, as enzymes are lacking here for their breakdown.

Stomach - The hydrolysis of starch, swallowed with amylase, is inhibited. The acidic environment of the stomach is not favorable for it.

The hydrolysis of proteins begins here, catalyzed by pepsin. Large protein molecules are broken down into peptides, fragments of the proteins.

Lipid molecules remain unchanged chemically, as there aren't enough enzymes for their hydrolysis.

Small Intestine - The hydrolysis of starch is resumed, catalyzed by the secretion of pancreatic amylase. Maltose, the product of this hydrolysis, is further degraded along with other disaccharides in the diet. The disaccharides and their monosaccharides produced by hydrolysis are:

maltose digested into glucose—the enzyme is maltase

sucrose digested into fructose and glucose—the enzyme is sucrase

lactose digested into galactose and glucose—the enzyme is lactase

Peptides are hydrolyzed into amino acids, step by step. Enzymes such as trypsin and chymotrypsin speed up this process. Amino acids are the subunits produced.

After the emulsification of fat globules by bile, fat molecules (triglycerides) are broken down into fatty acids and glycerol.

Problem Solving Example:

 What is the basic mechanism of digestion, and what digestive processes take place in the mouth and stomach?

 The process of digestion is the breakdown of large, ingested molecules into smaller, simple ones that can be absorbed and used by the body. The breakdown of these large molecules is called degradation. During degradation, some of the chemical bonds that hold

the large molecules together are split. The digestive enzymes cleave molecular bonds by a process called hydrolysis. In hydrolysis, a water molecule is added across the bond to cleave it.

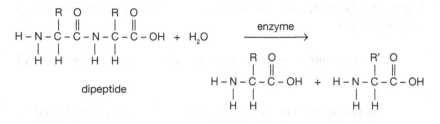

Hydrolysis of a dipeptide, R and R' represent different side chains

Within living systems, chemical reactions require specific enzymes to act as catalysts. Enzymes are very specific, acting only on certain substrates. In addition, different enzymes work best under unlike conditions. Digestive enzymes work best outside of the cell, for their optimum pHs lie either on the acidic (e.g., gastric enzymes) or basic (e.g., intestinal and pancreatic enzymes) side . The cell interior, however, requires an almost neutral (about 7.4) pH constantly. Digestive enzymes are secreted into the digestive tract by the cells that line or serve it.

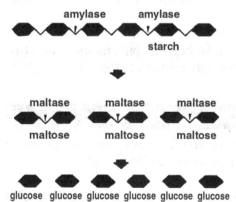

Digestion of a starch. Amylase in the saliva and in the pancreatic juice hydrolyzes the bonds between every other pair of glucose units, producing the disaccharide maltose. Maltose is digested to glucose by maltase, secreted by intestinal glands.

Digestion begins in the mouth. Most foods contain polysaccharides, such as starch, which are long chains of glucose molecules.

Saliva and the intestinal secretions contain enzymes that degrade such molecules. Salivary amylase, an enzyme that is also called ptyalin, hydrolyzes starch into maltose. (Compounds with names ending in "-ase" are enzymes, and those with the suffix "-ose" are sugars.) Glucose is eventually absorbed by the epithelial cells lining the small intestine.

The saliva has a pH of 6.5 to 6.8. This is the optimal range for salivary enzyme activity. Food spends a relatively short amount of time in the mouth, and eventually enters the stomach. The stomach is very acidic, with a pH of 1.5 to 2.5. The acid is secreted by special cells in the lining of the stomach called parietal cells. The low pH is required for the activity of the stomach enzyme pepsin. Rennin coagulates milk proteins in the infant's stomach, making them more susceptible to enzyme attack. Pepsin is a proteolytic enzyme (protease): it degrades proteins. Pepsin starts the protein digestion in the stomach by splitting the long proteins into shorter fragments, or peptides, that are further digested in the intestine. Pepsin will split any peptide bond involving the amino acids tyrosine or phenylalanine. There are 20 different kinds of amino acids that can make up a protein, and some proteins are thousands of amino acids long. The body needs the amino acids it obtains from digestion to synthesize its own proteins.

13.3.2 Motility/Secretion

Motility is the movement of the food mass through the tract, created by the contraction of the smooth muscle layer in the wall of the tract. By **secretion**, substances are introduced into the tract to prepare and digest the food. Several different hormones control these events.

Problem Solving Example:

 Explain how peristalsis moves food through the digestive tract.

 In each region of the digestive tract, rhythmic waves of constriction move food down the tract. This form of contractile activity is called peristalsis and involves involuntary smooth muscles. There are two layers of smooth muscle throughout most of the digestive tract. Circular muscles run around the circumference of the tract, while longitudinal muscles traverse its length.

Peristaltic waves passing over the stomach empty a small amount of material into the duodenum. Most of the material is forced back into the antrum.

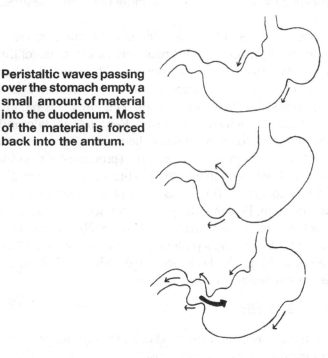

Once a food bolus is moved into the lower esophagus, circular muscles in the esophageal wall just behind the bolus contract, squeezing and pushing the food downward. At the same time, longitudinal muscles in the esophageal wall in front of the bolus relax to facilitate movement of the food. As the bolus moves, the muscles it passes also contract, so that a wave of contraction follows the bolus and constantly pushes it forward. This wave of constriction alternates with a wave of relaxation.

Swallowing initiates peristalsis, and once started, the waves of contraction cannot be stopped voluntarily. Like other involuntary responses, peristaltic waves are controlled by the autonomic nervous system. When a peristaltic wave reaches a sphincter, the sphincter opens slightly, and a small amount of food is forced through. Immediately afterwards, the sphincter closes to prevent the food from moving back. In the stomach, the waves of peristalsis increase in speed and intensity as they approach the pyloric end. As this happens, the pyloric sphincter of the stomach opens slightly. Some chyme escapes into the duodenum, but most of it is forced back into the stomach (see figure on the previous page). This allows the food to be more efficiently digested. There is little peristalsis in the intestine and more of a slower oscillating contraction. This is why most of the 12 to 24 hours that food requires for complete digestion is spent in the intestine.

Gastrin - It is secreted by endocrine cells in the wall of the stomach. The stomach is also the target organ. The secretion of gastrin is enhanced by the arrival of protein molecules from the diet. The hormone increases gastric (stomach) motility and the secretion of pepsin and HCl. These responses facilitate the digestion of proteins.

Enterogastrone - This hormone is secreted by endocrine cells in the wall of the small intestine when fat molecules arrive in this chamber. Enterogastrone signals the stomach to decrease motility and secretion. This is an appropriate response, as fat molecules require time to be processed and digested in the small intestine.

Secretin - Secreted by the small intestine, secretin signals the pancreas when food molecules arrive in this chamber. The pancreas responds with some enzymes and bicarbonate ions. The ions buffer the acidity of the arriving chyme, the partially digested food mass.

Cholecystokinin-pancreozymin (CCP) - Both of these hormones are secreted from the small intestine as food arrives. Cholecystokinin (CCK) signals the gallbladder to secrete more bile. Pancreozymin signals the pancreas to secrete more enzymes. All of these responses prepare and digest the food molecules.

Problem Solving Example:

  What controls the secretion of the digestive enzymes?

A Digestive enzyme secretion is regulated by two kinds of factors: neural and humoral (hormonal). Neural control is usually based upon the sensing of a physical mass of food. The stretching of the digestive tract (distension) is an example of this type of stimulation. It is interesting to note that most of the salivary and some of the gastric secretions are stimulated by smelling, tasting, and even thinking of food. Hormonal control, on the other hand, is much more specific. The presence of specific kinds of molecules in the ingested food stimulates receptor cells to produce their specific hormone. The hormone circulates in the blood until it reaches the secretory organs that it controls.

Activities of the Gastrointestinal Hormones

	Secretin	CCK	Gastrin
Secreted by:	Duodenum	Duodenum	Antrum of the stomach
Primary stimulus for hormone release	Acid in duodenum	Amino acids and fatty acids in duodenum	Peptides in stomach; Parasympathetic nerves to stomach
Effect on:			
Gastric motility	Inhibits	Inhibits	Stimulates
Gastric HCl secretion	Inhibits	Inhibits	STIMULATES *
Pancreatic secretion	Stimulates	Stimulates	Stimulates
Enzymes	Stimulates	STIMULATES *	Stimulates
Bile secretion	Stimulates	Stimulates	Stimulates
Gallbladder contraction	Stimulates	STIMULATES *	Stimulates
Intestinal juice secretion	Stimulates	Stimulates	

* Denotes that this hormone is quantitatively more important than the other two.

All secretory organs are under the influence of several factors. The presence of food in the mouth initiates gastric secretions by the stomach. When the food reaches the stomach, the distension of the stomach walls stimulates an increase in stomach motion and the partial production of gastrin. The hormone gastrin has several effects, the major of which is the stimulation of gastric juice secretion. It achieves this by stimulating gastric HCl secretion, which in turn induces protease activity. Pepsin, present in the gastric juice, cleaves proteins into many smaller chains. These small peptide chains stimulate receptor cells in the antrum of the stomach to produce more gastrin. Gastrin also has the ability to stimulate limited secretion in the intestine and pancreas. In addition, gastrin stimulates an increase in gastric motility and helps keep the sphincter of the esophagus tightly closed.

When partially digested food, or chyme, reaches the duodenum, its physical presence initiates peristalsis over the entire intestine. In addition, the acid in the chyme causes receptor cells to release the hormone secretin. Secretin has many functions. It slows down stomach motion and decreases gastric juice and gastrin production. This effectively keeps the food in the stomach for a longer period. At the same time, secretin prepares the intestine for neutralization of the acidic chyme by stimulating the release of alkaline bicarbonate ions in pancreatic juice.

Other receptor cells in the duodenum sense free amino acids and fats. These cells release a hormone called cholecystokinin or CCK, which stimulates the release of a pancreatic juice rich in digestive enzymes while slowing down the motion in the stomach. The more fat and protein there is in a meal, the longer digestion will occur. A review of the regulatory activities of gastrointestinal hormones is given in the accompanying table.

Note that CCK and secretin act synergistically. CCK stimulates secretion of a pancreatic juice rich in digestive enzymes, but it accentuates secretin's stimulation of a pancreatic juice rich in bicarbonate. Secretin stimulates secretion of a juice high in bicarbonate, but it accentuates CCK's secretion of a juice high in enzymes.

The control of secretions in digestion is a complex interaction of several factors. One's emotional state, as well as physical health, have a great influence on digestion. Age and diet are also critical factors. When a child is born, it does not have sufficient enzyme production to digest many foods other than milk. As we age, most adults stop producing rennin and lose the ability to fully digest milk. Humans have the most varied diet of all animals. This is reflected in the complex interactions of enzymes and hormones that control our digestion.

13.3.3 Absorption/Reabsorption/Excretion

The final products of hydrolysis in the small intestine are monosaccharides, amino acids, fatty acids, and glycerol. In addition, vitamins (e.g., A and C) and minerals (e.g., Na and Ca) move through the tract unaltered. These substances are absorbed through the mucosa, entering the capillaries of the submucosa. Most of these substances are transported by the hepatic portal system to the liver for further metabolism.

Reabsorption rates in the large intestine are high. If, for example, 9,000 ml of fluid are secreted throughout the tract over 24 hours, 8,900 ml can be reabsorbed by the body.

The remaining, unabsorbed material in the colon is eliminated from the body, under the control of various reflexes (gastrocolic reflex).

Problem Solving Examples:

Q The intestine, especially the small intestine, is a vital organ for absorption of nutrients required by the body. In what ways is it suitable for such a function?

A The small intestine is the region of the digestive tract between the stomach and the cecum. Its long, convoluted structure is an adaptation for absorption of nutrients. Structural modifications of the internal surfaces of the small intestine act to increase its surface area for absorption. First, the mucosa lining the intestine is thrown into numerous folds and ridges. Second, small finger-like projections called villi cover the entire surface of the mucosa (see figure). These villi are richly supplied with blood capillaries and lacteals (for absorption of fats) to facilitate absorption of nutrients. Third, individual epithelial cells lining the folds and villi have a "brush-border" on the surface facing the lumen, consisting of countless, closely packed, cylindrical processes known as microvilli. These microvilli add an enormous amount of surface area to that already present. The total internal surface area of the small intestine is thus incredibly large; this is advantageous for the purpose of absorption.

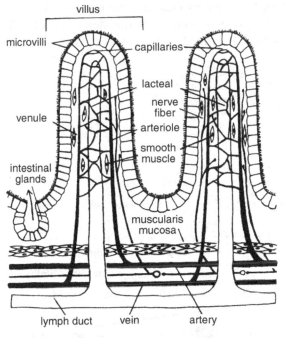

Structure of intestinal villi

The large intestine also has villi to increase its surface area. However, the number of villi present in the small intestine far exceeds that found in the large intestine. The main function of the large intestine is to absorb water from the undigested food substances and reduce the remains to a semisolid state before it is expelled through the anus.

 Discuss the absorption of glucose and amino acids. How does it differ from the mechanism of absorption of fatty acids?

Almost all the nutrient products obtained from digestion are absorbed through the walls of the small intestine. The total volume occupied by the small intestine is relatively small; however, the internal surface area of the small intestine is immense, allowing for very efficient absorption of digested nutrients. This large surface area is a result of the folds and ridges of the small intestine, compounded with the villi and microvilli that cover its internal surface. The villi are finger-like processes that extend into the lumen of the intestine. The microvilli are hair-like projections of the membrane of cells lining the villi. It is here that specific absorption takes place.

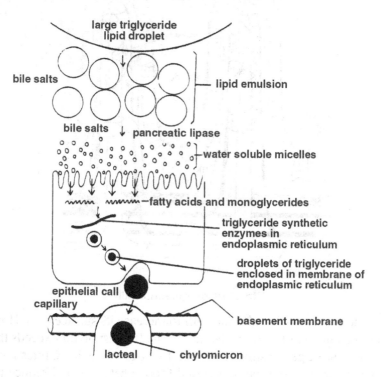

Summary of fat absorption across the walls of the small intestine

When glucose or free amino acids approach the cell membrane, they are bound by special groups of enzymes that are within the membrane. These enzymes quickly transport the molecules through the membrane into the cytoplasm. The nutrients are then transported across the intestinal epithelium into the blood. This occurs in part by simple diffusion, in part by facilitated diffusion, and in part by active transport. The presence of sodium in the lumen is required for monosaccharide transport. The various hexoses are absorbed by active transport. Amino acids are also absorbed by means of active transport. These nutrients are then circulated to the cells of the body, or transported to the liver for storage.

Glycerol and fatty acids are not selectively absorbed. After fats are digested in the intestinal lumen, the majority of their products, primarily fatty acids and monoglycerides, simply diffuse across the cell membrane because of their high solubility in membrane lipids. These are then brought into the endoplasmic reticulum (ER) of the epithelial cells, where they are resynthesized into triglycerides. These lipids, in turn, combine with specific proteins, forming lipoproteins. The lipoproteins aggregate into droplets called chylomicra within the ER. The ER then fuses with the cell surface and empties the chylomicra into the extracellular space. Here, they are absorbed by the lacteals of the lymphatic system and are eventually transferred into the bloodstream. After a high-fat meal, one's blood may become "milky looking," due to the high concentration of chylomicra. Note that no energy is required for fat absorption.

Another important aspect of absorption is the uptake of partially digested material. When disaccharides and dipeptides are within the vicinity of the cell membrane, the membrane extends itself, forming a pocket around the partially digested molecules. This pocket invaginates into the cell in a process known as pinocytosis. The pinocytotic vesicle fuses with another vesicle called a lysosome. The lysosome contains the cells own digestive enzymes. As these enzymes digest the vesicle's contents, the degraded nutrients diffuse through the membrane into the cytoplasm and are used by the cell.

Quiz: The Digestive System

1. The 10-inch body tube that accepts swallowed food is the

    (A) esophagus.

    (B) larynx.

    (C) nasal cavity.

    (D) pharynx.

    (E) trachea.

2. The function of bile salts is to

    (A) digest fat.

    (B) chemically degrade fat.

    (C) emulsify fat into smaller globules.

    (D) activate enzymes in pancreatic juice.

    (E) acidify a solution that the salt is in.

3. Which of the following is a protease?

    (A) Amylase

    (B) Maltose

    (C) Pepsin

    (D) Ptyalin

    (E) Sucrase

4. All of the following enzymes are involved in the digestion of food EXCEPT

    (A) pepsin.

    (B) trypsin.

    (C) maltase.

    (D) amylase.

    (E) ligase.

5. An exocrine gastric product that combines with vitamin B_{12} for absorption in the small intestine is

    (A) pepsin.

    (B) hydrochloric acid.

    (C) mucus.

    (D) intrinsic factor.

    (E) trypsin.

6. The last part of the human small intestine before entering the large intestine is the

    (A) cecum.   (D) ileum.

    (B) jejunum.   (E) pylorus.

    (C) duodenum.

7. The storage form of glucose is called

    (A) glycogen.   (D) dextrose.

    (B) glycine.   (E) sucrose.

    (C) glycerine.

8. A person afflicted with a complete obstruction of the common bile duct would have a decreased ability to digest

    (A) proteins.

    (B) carbohydrates.

    (C) nucleic acids.

    (D) fats.

    (E) None of the above.

9. Tying off the pancreatic ducts ties off

   (A) endocrine function.

   (B) neural function.

   (C) digestive function.

   (D) Both (A) and (B).

   (E) Both (B) and (C).

10. Ligation of the islets of Langerhans of the pancreas will deprive the circulatory system of

   (A) insulin.

   (B) trypsin.

   (C) serotonin.

   (D) bile.

   (E) pepsin.

ANSWER KEY

1.	(A)	6.	(D)
2.	(C)	7.	(A)
3.	(C)	8.	(D)
4.	(E)	9.	(C)
5.	(D)	10.	(A)

CHAPTER 14

The Renal System

14.1 Anatomy

The renal system consists of two **kidneys**, two **ureters**, one **urinary bladder**, and one **urethra**. Each kidney consists of over one million microscopic units called **nephrons**. The kidneys receive about 20 percent of the cardiac output every minute, so the collective action of the nephrons controls the composition of the extracellular fluid (ECF). Therefore, the kidneys make a major contribution to body chemistry and homeostasis. As they regulate the composition of the ECF, they produce urine.

14.1.1 Kidney

Each kidney is slightly above the waistline. The location of the kidney is retroperitoneal, meaning that it is posterior to the peritoneum, a serous membrane lining the abdominal cavity. Each kidney is between the peritoneum and the skeletal muscles of the dorsal body wall.

The size of the kidney is about 5 inches × 2 inches × 1 inch (length, width, thickness). A **renal artery** and **renal vein** enter it at its medial notch, the **hilum**.

Each kidney is bound by a thin, leathery **capsule**. Internally, this organ is composed of two layers. The outer **cortex** is reddish, with an abundant supply of blood vessels. The inner **medulla** consists of about one dozen **renal pyramids**. These wedges have a striated appearance.

Although the cortical tissue is mainly external, some of it does penetrate deeper into the kidney as **renal columns**. These columns alternate with the pyramids. The pointed ends of the pyramids, the **papillae**, project deep and medially into the kidney. Each papilla fits into a funnel-like structure, the **calyx**. All of these calyces converge into a deep, medial cavity called the **renal pelvis**.

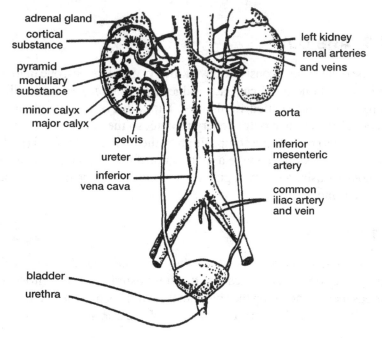

The human renal system seen from the ventral right side. The right kidney is shown cut open to reveal internal structures.

14.1.2 Other Organs

The **ureter** is a tube, 10 to 12 inches long, that extends from the pelvis of the kidney. This muscular tube propels the urine into the **urinary bladder** by peristalsis. The bladder, located in the pelvic cavity, stores the urine.

When the bladder becomes filled with urine, a reflex (micturition reflex) leads to a contraction of the smooth muscle layer in its wall. This forces urine out of the bladder and through the **urethra**. This is the final passageway of the urinary tract, which is inferior to the bladder. If two sphincter muscles in the urethra relax as the bladder contracts, urine is eliminated from the bladder.

14.1.3 Nephron

The nephron is made up of a **renal corpuscle** plus several regions of **tubules**.

The renal corpuscle of this microscopic unit consists of the **glomerulus** (a ball of capillaries) and a double-walled cup (**Bowman's capsule**). The renal corpuscle is the site of **filtration**, the passage of plasma substances from the glomerulus into the Bowman's capsule.

From the renal artery, a series of arteries and smaller vessels send blood into each glomerulus. An **afferent arteriole** sends blood into the glomerulus directly. An **efferent arteriole** transports blood away from the glomerulus. The efferent vessel breaks down into a second set of capillaries, the **peritubular capillaries**. They surround the tubular portion of the nephron.

The tubular portion of the nephron has four main regions. Filtrate from Bowman's capsule first passes into the **proximal convoluted tubule** in the cortex. Next, the filtrate enters **Henle's loop** (also known as the loop of Henle), first through its descending limb and then through its ascending limb. This loop extends deep into the medulla. From there, fluid enters the **distal convoluted tubule**, also in the cortex. From that tubule, fluid passes into the **collecting duct** which passes deep into the medulla.

After filtration, fluid in the tubules of the nephrons undergoes two more processes, both involving the peritubular capillaries: **tubular reabsorption** and **tubular secretion**. Some blood is not filtered and passes into the efferent vessels and peritubular capillaries. Many substances that are filtered are returned to the peritubular capillaries from the tubules by reabsorption, often at high rates (e.g., water, glucose). The blood in the peritubular capillaries collects into other vessels that join the renal vein, the last vessel draining the organ.

Problem Solving Example:

Q In humans, the kidney performs the bulk of the excretion of wastes from the body. Outline the structure of the human kidney and urinary system.

A Located on each posterior side of the human body just below the level of the stomach are the bean-shaped kidneys. Each kidney is about 10 cm long, and consists of three parts: an outer layer called the cortex, an inner layer called the medulla, and a sac-like chamber called the renal pelvis (see figure on the next page). The functional unit of a kidney is the nephron; there are about a million nephrons in each kidney. A nephron consists of two components: a tubule for conducting noncellular fluid and a capillary network for carrying blood cells and plasma. The mechanisms by which the kidneys perform their functions depend on both the physical and physiological relationships between these two components of the nephron.

Throughout its course, the kidney tubule is composed of a single layer of epithelial cells that differs in structure and function from one portion of the tubule to another. The blind end of the tubule is Bowman's capsule, a sac embedded in the cortex and lined with thin epithelial cells. The curved side of Bowman's capsule is in intimate contact with the glomerulus, a compact tuft of branching blood capillaries, while the other opens into the first portion of the tubular system called the proximal convoluted tubule. The proximal convoluted tubule leads to a portion of the tubule known as the loop of Henle. This hairpin loop consists of a descending and an ascending limb, both of which extend into the medulla. Following the loop, the tubule once more becomes coiled as the distal convoluted tubule. Finally, the tubule runs a straight course as the collecting duct. From the glomerulus to the beginning of the collecting duct, each of the million or so nephrons is completely separate from its neighbors. However, the collecting ducts from sepa-

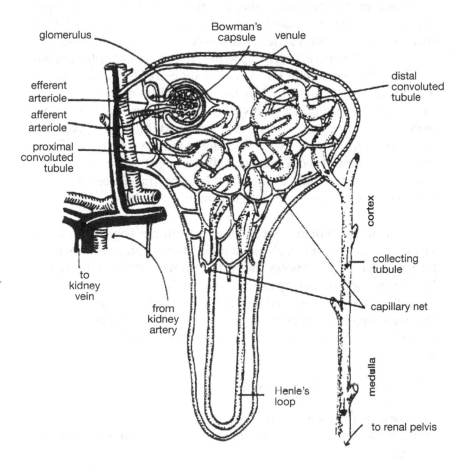

Diagram of a single nephron and its blood vessels

rate nephrons join to form common ducts, which in turn join to form even longer ducts, which finally empty into a large central cavity, the renal pelvis, at the base of each kidney. The renal pelvis is continuous with the ureter, which empties into the urinary bladder where urine is temporarily stored. The urine remains unchanged in the bladder, and when eventually excreted, has the same composition as when it left the collecting ducts.

Blood enters the kidney through the renal artery, which upon reaching the kidney divides into smaller and smaller branches. Each small artery gives off a series of arterioles, each of which leads to a glomerulus. The arterioles leading to the glomerulus are called afferent arterioles. The glomerulus protrudes into the cup of Bowman's capsule and is completely surrounded by the epithelial lining of the capsule. The functional significance of this anatomical arrangement is that blood in the capillaries of the glomerulus is separated from the space within Bowman's capsule only by two extremely thin layers: (1) the single-celled capillary wall and (2) the one-celled lining of Bowman's capsule. This thin barrier permits the filtration of plasma (the noncellular blood fraction) from the capillaries into Bowman's capsule.

Ordinarily, capillaries recombine to form the beginnings of the venous system. However, glomerular capillaries instead recombine to form another set of arterioles, called the efferent arterioles. Soon after leaving the region of the capsule, these arterioles branch again, forming a capillary network surrounding the tubule. Each excretory tubule is thus well supplied with circulatory vessels. The capillaries eventually rejoin to form venous channels, through which the blood ultimately leaves the kidney.

14.2 Renal Physiology

The nephrons carry out three processes that regulate the composition of the extracellular fluid and form the urine: **filtration**, **reabsorption**, and **secretion**.

14.2.1 Filtration

Filtration is the first step of renal physiology. By filtration, substances leave the blood plasma, passing from the glomerulus into the Bowman's capsule. Large amounts of most substances (e.g., water, glucose, sodium) are filtered. The one exception is the plasma proteins, as these molecules are too large to pass through the pores in the walls of the glomerulus. Therefore, they do not leave the blood.

The filtrate is produced by an interaction of several pressures. **Blood pressure** is the major one, tending to force substances from the capillary into the capsule. For a capillary it is abnormally high at the glomerulus. One example is 70 mmHg.

Two pressures oppose the blood pressure, as they are responsible for the movement of substances in the opposite direction. A **capsular pressure** in Bowman's capsule forces fluid back into the blood. By a **colloidal osmotic pressure** (COP), fluid is drawn into the blood by osmosis. The blood in the glomerulus remains hypertonic because the plasma proteins, colloids based on their size, are not forced out of the capillary by the blood pressure.

If the capsular pressure and COP are 20 and 30, respectively, as examples, the blood pressure forcing substances out of the blood is still greater. The difference between the blood pressure and the two pressures opposing it yields a net pressure, the **effective filtration pressure** (EFP):

$$EFP = 70 - (20 + 30) = 20$$

In this example, a net pressure of 20 units forces plasma substances into the blood of the glomerulus.

Filtration is a nonselective process, as all plasma substances (except the plasma proteins) pass from the blood plasma into the capsule in significant quantities. The cells of the blood are also not normally filtered.

Filtered substances next pass from the Bowman's capsule into the proximal convoluted tubule of the nephron.

Problem Solving Example:

 With reference to fluid pressures, explain the mechanism underlying glomerular filtration.

A The mean blood pressure in the large arteries of the body is approximately 100 mmHg. However, as the blood passes through the arterioles connecting the renal artery to the glomeruli, the blood pressure decreases so that the pressure in the glomerular capillaries is usually only about half the mean arterial pressure or 50 mmHg. This level is considerably higher than in other capillaries of the body, due to the fact that the arterioles leading to the glomeruli are wider than most other arterioles and therefore offer less resistance to flow. The force driving fluid out of the glomerulus and into Bowman's capsule is the pressure of the blood in the glomerular capillaries. But this hydrostatic pressure favoring filtration is not completely unopposed. There is fluid within Bowman's capsule, resulting in a capsular hydrostatic pressure of about 10 mmHg, which resists the flow into the capsule. The presence of protein in the plasma and its absence in Bowman's capsule results in a second force opposing filtration. This difference in protein concentration between the capsule and the blood induces an osmotic flow of water into the blood. This osmotic pressure, also known as colloidal osmotic pressure, equals roughly 30 mmHg.

Summing the forces, there is a glomerular capillary blood pressure of 50 mmHg favoring filtration, a 10 mmHg opposition to filtration due to fluid in Bowman's capsule, and a 30 mmHg pressure working against filtration due to a protein concentration difference between the blood and the capsule fluid, resulting in a net glomerular filtration pressure of 10 mmHg. This net pressure forces fluid from the blood into Bowman's capsule.

14.2.2 Reabsorption

Most filtered substances are returned to the blood by the second step of renal function, reabsorption. Specifically, substances pass from the tubules of the nephron into the blood of the peritubular capillaries.

Usually, reabsorption occurs at high percentage rates. For example, if 190 liters of water are filtered over 24 hours, around 189 liters of water can be reabsorbed. Therefore, the rate of reabsorption for water is over 99 percent. Normally the reabsorption rate of glucose is 100 percent. If 300 grams of glucose are filtered over 24 hours, all 300 grams are usually reabsorbed.

If a substance is not secreted, a possible last step of renal physiology, the amount of a substance eliminated is equal to the amount filtered minus the amount reabsorbed. The amount that is not reabsorbed does not reenter the blood. It will remain in the tubules of the nephron and be eliminated. As one example:

190 liters of water filtered – 189 liters reabsorbed = 1 liter eliminated

Unlike filtration, reabsorption is a very selective process. Substances are returned to the blood to the degree they are needed for body metabolism. To fulfill this need, reabsorption is controlled.

Sodium reabsorption is controlled by **aldosterone**, a hormone secreted by the nearby adrenal cortex. If more sodium is needed, more aldosterone is secreted. It signals the nephron tubules, particularly cells in the wall of the proximal convoluted tubules, to transport more sodium back into the blood. If less sodium is needed by the body, less aldosterone is secreted to stimulate sodium reabsorption.

The reabsorption of water depends on the reabsorption of sodium at the proximal convoluted tubule. The reabsorption of water there is **obligatory**. This means that it must occur. The blood in the peritubular capillaries becomes hypertonic as it accumulates reabsorbed sodium. The tubular wall is permeable to water that follows sodium ions by osmosis. This accounts for a large amount of the total reabsorption of water.

The reabsorption of water also affects blood pressure. Water reabsorption adds more fluid to the vessels. Just as more water in a garden hose increases its pressure, adding more fluid to blood vessels increases their pressure. Cells in the juxtaglomerular apparatus, cells near the afferent vessel, detect blood pressure changes. These cells secrete **renin**, an enzyme that converts the plasma protein angiotensinogen into **angiotensin**.

Angiotensin signals the adrenal cortex to secrete aldosterone, which stimulates sodium and water reabsorption. One example of this chain of events occurs to oppose blood pressure if it decreases:

blood pressure decreases, renin increases, angiotensin increases, aldosterone increases, sodium reabsorption increases, water reabsorption increases, blood pressure increases

In the distal convoluted tubules and collecting ducts, the reabsorption of water is **facultative**, meaning it varies and is not obligatory. A small amount of water can be reabsorbed near the end of the nephron, depending on signaling from the hormone **ADH** (antidiuretic hormone). If more water is needed, more ADH is secreted from the posterior lobe of the pituitary. Therefore, on the output side, more water is reabsorbed and less is eliminated in the urine.

The **hypothalamus** senses the solute concentration of the blood and signals the posterior lobe to make this final adjustment of reabsorption. The hypothalamus also has a thirst center that controls water intake by drinking. If the blood is too hypertonic, one example that restores a balance is:

Hypertonic blood means more water needed in ECF (blood) to dilute the solutes in the blood. The hypothalamus senses this condition and more ADH is secreted. More water is reabsorbed and less is eliminated. In addition, the sense of thirst increases and adds water on the input side.

Cells composing the walls of the nephron are specialized to carry out unique functions. The cells of the proximal convoluted tubule have microvilli, establishing a brush border. This increases their surface area for reabsorption.

Cells in the ascending limb in the loop of Henle have numerous mitochondria. These organelles, or powerplants, give the ascending cells the energy to pump sodium back into the fluid surrounding the descending limb. This makes the surrounding fluid more hypertonic. This leads to the greater reabsorption of water as it leaves the tubule by osmosis when passing through the wall of the descending limb.

Most filtered substances have an upper limit, or threshold, over which they cannot be reabsorbed. Glucose, for example, normally has a 100 percent reabsorption rate. However, at concentrations over 180 mg/100 ml in the filtrate, the tubule cells lack the time or energy to return the extra levels of glucose into the blood.

In the blood and filtrate of a person with diabetes mellitus, the blood sugar level can be very high (e.g., 1,200 mg/100 ml). The extra glucose that cannot be reabsorbed will be eliminated in the urine. A normal level of sugar in the blood and filtrate (e.g., 100 mg/100 ml) can be controlled by normal renal functions and completely reabsorbed.

14.2.3 Secretion

Some substances undergo a third process called secretion. By this process, substances are transported from the blood in the peritubular capillaries into the nephrons near their ends—the distal convoluted tubules and collecting ducts. Potassium ions, which are usually reabsorbed at a rate of 100 percent, may be added back to the nephron by this third step. Hydrogen ions are often secreted to eliminate them from the blood. This opposes their buildup in the blood, a condition called acidosis.

The secretion of hydrogen supplements buffer systems in the blood. Buffers are chemicals that react with free hydrogen ions in the blood and eliminate them by making them parts of other compounds. For example, the buffer compound sodium bicarbonate reacts with free hydrogen ions to produce this effect.

If a molecule such as urea (nitrogen waste product) is filtered and not reabsorbed, it will be eliminated from the body by passing through the following structures:

renal artery, other arteries, afferent arteriole, glomerulus, proximal convoluted tubule, loop of Henle (descending limb), loop of Henle (ascending limb), distal convoluted tubule, collecting duct, renal papilla, calyx, pelvis, ureter, bladder, urethra

Numerous collecting ducts converge at the papilla end of each pyramid of the medulla. From here, the funnel-like calyces accept molecules that will enter the larger structures of the renal system for elimination.

Problem Solving Example:

Q There are three processes that enable the kidney to remove wastes while conserving the useful components of the blood. What are these processes, and where do they occur?

A Blood flowing to the kidneys first undergoes glomerular filtration. This occurs at the junction of the glomerular capillaries and the wall of Bowman's capsule. The blood plasma is filtered as it passes through the capillaries, which are freely permeable to water and solutes of small molecular dimension yet relatively impermeable to large molecules, especially the plasma proteins. Water, salts, glucose, urea, and other small molecules pass from the blood into the cavity of Bowman's capsule to become the glomerular filtrate.

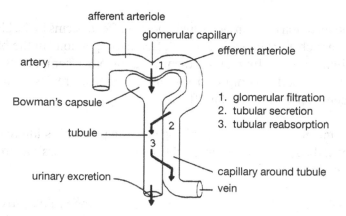

Three basic components of renal function

It has been demonstrated that the filtrate in Bowman's capsule contains virtually no protein and that all low weight crystalloids (glucose, protons, chloride ions, etc.) are present in the same concentrations as in plasma.

If it were not for the process of tubular reabsorption, the composition of the urine would be identical to that of the glomerular filtrate. This would be extremely wasteful, since a great deal of water, glucose, amino acids, and other useful substances present in the filtrate would be lost. Tubular reabsorption is strictly defined as the transfer of material from the tubular lumen back to the blood through the walls of the capillary network in intimate contact with the tubule. The principal portion of the tubule involved in reabsorption is the proximal convoluted tubule. This tubule is lined with epithelial cells having many hair-like processes extending into its lumen. These processes are the chief sites of tubular reabsorption. As the filtrate passes through the tubule, the epithelial cells reabsorb much of the water and virtually all the glucose, amino acids, and other substances useful to the body. The cells then secrete these back into the bloodstream. The secretion of these substances into the blood is accomplished against a concentration gradient, and is thus an energy-consuming process—one using ATP. The rates at which substances are reabsorbed, and therefore the rates at which wastes are excreted (because what is not reabsorbed is eliminated), are constantly subjected to physiological control. The ability to vary the excretion of water, sodium, potassium, hydrogen, calcium, phosphate ions, and many other substances is the essence of the kidney's ability to regulate the internal environment. Reabsorption also occurs in the distal convoluted tubules, where sodium is actively reabsorbed under the influence of aldosterone, a hormone secreted by the adrenal cortex. When this occurs, chloride passively follows due to an electrochemical gradient; water is also reabsorbed because of an osmotic gradient established by the reabsorption of sodium and chloride. In addition, reabsorption of water takes place in the distal convoluted tubule and collecting duct, stimulated by the posterior pituitary hormone vasopressin, also known as antidiuretic hormone (ADH). ADH increases the permeability of the distal convoluted tubule and collecting duct to water, allowing water to leave the lumen of the nephron and render the urine more concentrated.

The kidney also removes wastes by means of tubular secretion. This process involves the movement of additional waste materials directly from the bloodstream into the lumen of the tubules, without passing through Bowman's capsule. Tubular secretion may be either active or passive; that is, it may or may not require energy. Of the large number of different substances transported into the tubules by tubular secretion, only a few are normally found in the body. The most important of these are potassium and hydrogen ions. Most other substances secreted are foreign substances, such as penicillin. In some animals, like the toadfish, whose kidneys lack glomeruli and Bowman's capsules, secretion by the tubules is the only method available for excretion.

Quiz: The Renal System

1. The process by which blood plasma moves out of the glomerulus capillaries and into Bowman's capsule is called

    (A) reabsorption.

    (B) secretion.

    (C) countercurrent exchange.

    (D) filtration.

    (E) multiplication.

2. The subunit of a kidney that purifies blood and maintains a safe balance of solutes and water in humans is called

    (A) glomerulus.

    (B) loop of Henle.

    (C) urethra.

    (D) Bowman's capsule.

    (E) nephron.

3. The permeability of the walls of the distal convoluted collecting tubules of the kidneys to water is regulated by

    (A) the amount of water.

    (B) the concentration of salts.

    (C) vasopressin.

    (D) the adrenals.

    (E) the thymus.

4. Which of the following statements incorrectly describe(s) the functions and/or characteristics of nephrons in the human kidney?

    (A) Active transport of Na^+ ions.

    (B) Passive transport of Na^+ ions.

    (C) The walls of the ascending limb of loop of Henle must be watertight.

    (D) The urine in the distal convoluted tubule is less concentrated than the initial filtrate.

    (E) None of the above.

5. The functional unit of the human excretory system is the

    (A) kidney.

    (B) nephron.

    (C) glomerulus.

    (D) urinary bladder.

    (E) urethra.

6. When the blood of an individual becomes hypertonic, the kidney will then

    (A) secrete more antidiuretic hormone (ADH).

    (B) excrete more water.

    (C) decrease its rate of filtration.

    (D) excrete a smaller volume of more concentrated urine.

    (E) increase its rate of filtration.

7. The walls of the collecting ducts and distal convoluted tubule are made permeable to water by

    (A) aldosterone.

    (B) parathormone.

    (C) luteinizing hormone (LH).

    (D) antidiuretic hormone (ADH).

    (E) calcitonin.

8. The hydrostatic pressure of the blood within the glomerular capillaries is

    (A) less than the mean blood pressure in the large arteries of the body.

    (B) about half the mean arterial pressure.

    (C) usually about 50 mmHg.

    (D) All of the above.

    (E) None of the above.

9. The process whereby urea is removed from blood in the glomerulus is known as

   (A) tubular secretion.   (D) osmosis.

   (B) reabsorption.   (E) active transport.

   (C) ultrafiltration.

10. The thin barrier at Bowman's capsule allows for filtration of

    (A) whole blood.

    (B) ammonia.

    (C) plasma.

    (D) oxygen.

    (E) urine.

ANSWER KEY

1.	(D)	6.	(D)
2.	(E)	7.	(D)
3.	(C)	8.	(D)
4.	(E)	9.	(C)
5.	(B)	10.	(C)

CHAPTER 15

The Reproductive System

The male and female reproductive systems produce sex cells. In addition, the female system provides the internal environment for fertilization and for the development of the embryo and fetus.

15.1 Male Reproductive System

The male reproductive system consists of the pair of testes (singular, testis), ducts, glands, and external genitalia.

Testis - Each testis, an oval-shaped structure, is suspended in the sac-like **scrotum**. The testis is encased by a fibrous capsule, the **tunica albuginea**. The dense fibrous tissue of this capsule continues internally as a series of **septa** or walls. These walls subdivide the interior of each testis into a number of **lobules** or chambers. Each lobule contains **seminiferous tubules** and **interstitial cells** (**cells of Leydig**).

The seminiferous tubules are the site of **spermatogenesis**, sperm cell production. The tubules from each lobule converge and join posteriorly at the **rete testis**. The rete testis connects to the **epididymis**, a long structure, next to each testis posteriorly. The **vas deferens**, a major duct of the male reproductive tract, exits from the base of each epididymis.

The interstitial cells produce and secrete the hormone **testosterone**. This substance promotes the development of the male reproductive organs and secondary male characteristics (e.g., pitch of voice, hair growth on the face).

Ducts - The ducts form a connected series of passageways for the migration of sperm cells when they are ejaculated. This series of ducts forms the male reproductive tract.

The **epididymis** is a site where sex cells are stored and where they mature. Each **vas deferens (ductus deferens)**, along with blood vessels and nerves, is part of a **spermatic cord**. From each side of the scrotum, this combination of structures passes through the **inguinal canal**, a passageway leading from the scrotum into the pelvic cavity. The vas deferens conducts ejaculated sperm cells into this cavity.

From its ascent into the pelvic cavity, each vas deferens approaches the bladder from the anterior side. It passes over the top and descends on the posterior side, medial to where each ureter enters the bladder. The expanded end of the vas deferens is the **ampulla**. The two ampullae join, forming the **common ejaculatory duct**. This single structure passes through the **prostate gland**, which is inferior to the bladder. Within this gland, the common ejaculatory duct joins the **urethra**.

The urethra has three regions. The **prostatic urethra** is the first region, exiting from the bladder. From the point where the prostatic urethra merges with the common ejaculatory duct, the urinary and reproductive systems of the male are served by a common tract. The **membranous urethra** is a short region after the prostatic urethra, but before the tract enters the penis. The **penile urethra** is the last region, passing through the cavernous (spacious) tissue of the penis.

Glands - Several glands add seminal fluid to sperm cells migrating through the male tract. Semen is the mixture of sperm cells and seminal fluid formed by this addition.

The **epididymis** is a part of the tract, storing cells from the testis before they enter the vas deferens. It also adds a small percentage of the seminal fluid.

A pair of **seminal vesicles** add about 60 percent of the seminal fluid. Each gland secretes fluid into the ampulla of the vas deferens. The single, large **prostate gland** adds about 30 percent of the seminal fluid to the prostatic urethra. A pair of **Cowper's** (**bulbourethral**) glands add a small amount of fluid to the urethra as it passes into the posterior part of the penis.

External Genitalia - The **scrotum** is covered with skin externally. This structure is made up of two sacs separated by a septum. Each sac houses one testis, epididymis, and the beginning of each spermatic cord.

The **penis** contains three masses of cavernous tissue. This tissue has spaces that can fill with blood, causing the penis to become erect. More blood enters the penis when arteries serving this organ dilate, producing an erection. The two large **corpora cavernosa** (singular, corpus cavernosum) are separated by a septum. The **corpus spongiosum** surrounds the urethra. It expands into the **glans**, the blunt and enlarged end of the penis.

15.2 Female Reproductive System

The female reproductive system consists of a pair of ovaries and two uterine tubes, plus the uterus and vagina. The external genitalia are also part of this system.

Ovary - Each ovary is attached to the broad ligament, a fan-shaped structure that is posterior to the uterus and oviducts. The pair of ovaries stores nearly a half million immature sex cells. During ovulation, one sex cell matures and is released from the ovary into the oviduct. The ovaries also secrete changing levels of two hormones, **estrogen** and **progesterone**, during each female reproductive cycle.

Oviduct - On each side of the body, the expanded end of the oviduct (**uterine tube, Fallopian tube**) curves over the ovary. At its opposite end, the oviduct enters the fundus, the superior region of the uterus. A sex cell released from the ovary during ovulation enters the oviduct, drawn in by the muscular contractions of this part of the female reproductive tract. Normally, when a cell is fertilized, the process occurs in the oviduct, becoming an embryo of about 200 cells by the time it arrives in the cavity of the uterus.

Uterus - The uterus resembles an inverted triangle. The **fundus** is the dome-shaped region. The **body** is inferior to the fundus, tapering into a **cervix**. The cervix is the most inferior region, which fits into the vagina.

The uterus has three layers. The **endometrium** is a mucous membrane that lines the cavity of this organ. It is the site where the embryo implants after arriving from the uterine tube. It develops a vascular and glandular makeup to receive and maintain this early stage of development. The **myometrium** is the middle layer of smooth muscle. Its contraction during labor expels the fetus during parturition (birth). The **epimetrium** is a serous membrane that lines most of the external surface.

The uterus provides the internal environment for the prenatal development of the embryo and fetus.

Vagina - The vagina is the organ of copulation, a four- to six-inch muscular tube that accepts the penis. **Bartholin (vestibular) glands** at its external opening secrete substances that serve as lubricants for this process.

External Genitalia - The external genitalia consist of a pair of **labia majora**, which are external folds that are lateral to the pair of medial **labia minora**. These medial folds unite anteriorly to form a small mass of erectile tissue, the **clitoris**. Posteriorly, these folds unite to form the **posterior fourchette**. Within the labia minora, the opening of the urethra is anterior to the opening of the vagina.

The **vestibule** is the region extending from the clitoris to the posterior fourchette. The **mon pubis** is an elevated region that is anterior to the vestibule.

Problem Solving Example:

Q Trace the path of the sperm from the testes to its union with the egg in the human.

A In order to trace this path, we must first outline some aspects of the human male and female reproductive systems, illustrated in the figures below and on the next page. In normal males, the testes lie in the scrotum, a sac attached to the lower anterior wall of the abdomen. The testes reside in the body cavity during early embryonic development, but before birth they descend into the cavities of the scrotum. The inguinal canals are connections between the scrotum and body cavity; these canals are blocked off by connective tissue after the testes descend. The testes are located in the scrotal sacs because the sperm within them require cooler temperatures than the internal body temperature in order to survive and mature.

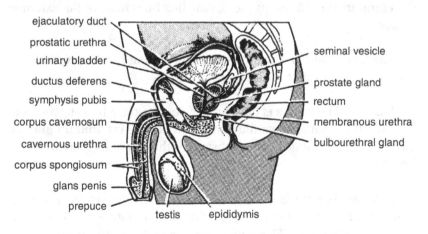

Reproductive system of the human male, lateral view

Each testis consists of roughly 1,000 coiled tubules called seminiferous tubules. It is in these tubules that the germ cells produce the sperm. Sertoli cells are also present and nourish the developing sperm. Connected to the seminiferous tubules via fine tubes called vasa efferentia is the epididymis, which is a single, complexly coiled tube in which sperm are stored and mature. The epididymis, which is derived from the embryonic kidney, empties into the vas deferens. This duct passes from the scrotum through the inguinal canal into the abdominal cavity, over the urinary bladder to a point where it opens into the ejaculatory duct, which empties into the urethra, the duct that leads from the urinary bladder to the exterior. Thus, in the male, the urethra serves as a common passageway for both reproductive and excretory functions. The urethra passes through the penis and is flanked by three columns of erectile tissue. This tissue becomes enlarged with blood during periods of sexual excitement, causing the penis to become erect. The engorgement of the penis is caused by arterial dilation and increased blood flow at unchanged arterial pressure. Prior to ejaculation, sperm from the testes pass through the vasa efferentia into the epididymis. During ejaculation, sperm from the epididymis are moved through the vas deferens by peristaltic contractions of its walls. Fluids are added to the sperm at the time of ejaculation. These fluids come from three pairs of glands: the seminal vesicles, the prostate glands (which in the human are fused into a single gland), and Cowper's bulbourethral glands. The mixture of secretions from these three sets of glands is termed seminal fluid. Semen consists of the sperm and seminal fluid. The seminal fluid consists of mucus (from seminal and bulbourethral secretions) and nutrients (seminal secretions), in a milky alkaline fluid (prostatic secretions).

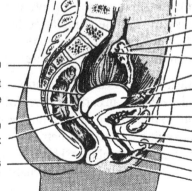

Reproductive system of the human female, lateral view

During copulation, the male's penis is inserted into the female's vagina, and semen is released there. Surrounding the vagina are the labia majora, two folds of fatty tissue covered by skin richly endowed with hair and sebaceous glands. These folds extend dorsally and down, enclosing the openings of the urethra and the vagina and merging behind them. The labia minora—thin folds of tissue devoid of hair—lie within the folds of the labia majora and are usually concealed by them. At the ventral junction of these two is the clitoris, a sensitive, erectile organ, which is the major site of female sexual excitement. The external female sex organs are collectively known as the vulva.

The vagina is a single, muscular tube that extends from the exterior to the uterus. From the vagina, the sperm swim, by motion of their flagella, through the cervix, the muscular ring of the uterus that projects into the vagina, and pass into the uterus. From there, they enter the Fallopian tubes (also known as the oviducts) where one may fertilize the secondary oocyte, if it is present. If fertilization does occur, the oocyte completes the second meiotic division, and the zygote (fertilized egg) is formed. Cleavage of the zygote begins in the Fallopian tube and will have proceeded to a multicellular state by the time the egg enters into the uterus and is implanted.

15.3 Female Reproductive Cycle

The events of the female reproductive cycle are controlled by the interaction of many hormones: follicle stimulating hormone (FSH), luteinizing hormone (LH), estrogen, and progesterone. Over a 28-day cycle, used here as an example, the major events are:

1. During **menstruation** there is a disintegration and loss of the endometrium. This occurs if an early embryo does not enter the uterus and implant to the inner lining. In this case the vascular and glandular thickening of the endometrium is not necessary to accept and maintain the embryo. The concentration of all hormones is low through this period. Menstruation can last over the first five days.

2. The secretion of **FSH**, from the **anterior lobe** of the **pituitary gland**, increases early in the cycle. FSH eventually stimulates the development of an **ovarian follicle**, a layer of cells surrounding one female sex cell in one of the ovaries. This event signals the onset of the **follicular phase**, the stage of the cycle after menstruation.

3. Cells of the active ovarian follicle secrete increased amounts of **estrogen**.

4. The surge in estrogen stimulates a proliferation of the endometrial lining, causing it to thicken.

5. By negative feedback, the increase of estrogen produces a gradual decrease in FSH, probably by signaling the hypothalamus that, in turn, controls the anterior lobe.

6. As FSH is gradually decreasing, the secretion of **LH** is gradually increasing. Peak levels of LH produce ovulation. This event occurs at about 14 days before the beginning of the next cycle. In a 28-day cycle, this is the midpoint. At this midpoint, the follicle is converted to the **corpus luteum**.

7. The conversion to the corpus luteum signals the beginning of the **luteal phase**. This stage takes up about the last half of the entire cycle. Initially in this phase the corpus luteum is maintained by LH.

8. The corpus luteum secretes increased levels of **progesterone** immediately after ovulation.

9. Increased progesterone, plus a new surge in estrogen secretion several days into the luteal phase, produces further maintenance and development of the endometrium.

10. The increase in progesterone and estrogen also feeds back to the hypothalamus to diminish the level of LH as the luteal phase progresses.

11. As LH drops off through the luteal phase, the corpus luteum cannot be maintained. It gradually degenerates, leading to a decrease in estrogen and progesterone during the final days of the luteal phase.

12. As estrogen and progesterone drop off by the end of the cycle, the endometrium is no longer maintained. It begins to disintegrate, leading to menstruation and the onset of the next cycle.

If fertilization and implantation occur, the endometrium does not degenerate. When implantation occurs, the woman becomes pregnant. Estrogen and progesterone levels remain high, supporting the development of the embryo and fetus. The production of an additional hormone, the **human chorionic gonadotropin** (HCG) also supports the development of the embryo and fetus. Some of this hormone is excreted in the urine. Its detection by testing a urine sample is the basis for the pregnancy test.

Problem Solving Example:

Q The female menstrual cycle lasts roughly 28 days. Trace the ovarian and hormonal changes that occur during a normal menstrual cycle.

A Under the influence of primarily FSH from the pituitary, a single ovarian follicle containing an ovum reaches maturity in about two weeks. During the second week the follicle cells and other ovarian cell types are stimulated by FSH to increase their secretion of estrogen. Near the middle of the cycle, or about the 14th day, the heightened level of estrogen in the blood reaches a critical value that stimulates the hypothalamus to signal the pituitary to release a surge of LH. This surge of LH induces rupture of the ovarian follicle. This releases the mature ovum into the Fallopian tube of the uterus, a process called ovulation. Estrogen secretion decreases for several days following ovulation, perhaps because of the negative feedback effect of excess estrogen on FSH, which stimulates its production. The ruptured follicle is rapidly transformed into the corpus luteum, which secretes progesterone and,

Female Reproductive Cycle

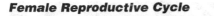

hypothalamus	FSH stimulating center more active			LH stimulating center more active	
anterior pituitary	FSH		LH		
ovary	follicle	ovulation		corpus luteum	
			Progesterone		
		Estrogen			
uterine lining			thickness of uterine lining		
days	2 4 flow phase (5)	6 8 10 12 follicular phase (9)	16 18 20 22 24 26 luteal phase (14)		30 flow phase

The sequence of events in the 28-day human menstrual cycle

in lesser amounts, estrogen. The estrogen secreted by the corpus luteum raises its level in the blood, which inhibits further FSH secretion. Progesterone suppresses additional LH production, and thus prevents additional ovulation from occurring. The combined influence of progesterone and estrogen thickens and prepares the uterus for implantation of the embryo (in the event of fertilization). Failure of oocyte fertilization leads to the degeneration of the corpus luteum during the last few days of the cycle. The disintegrating corpus luteum is unable to maintain its secretion of estrogen and progesterone, and their blood concentrations drop rapidly. The marked decrease of estrogen and progesterone leads to degeneration of the uterine wall followed by sloughing off of the uterine surface tissue. It also results in the removal of inhibition of FSH secretion, ovum development is stimulated, and the cycle begins anew.

The cycle is usually broken up into four general phases. The first phase, encompassing follicle development up to ovulation, is called the follicular phase and lasts about nine days. FSH and estrogen dominate during the phase. The second phase, lasting from ovulation until the beginning of the disintegration of the uterine lining, is called the luteal phase and lasts approximately 14 days. Progesterone dominates during this phase. Following this phase is the flow phase, which lasts five days and is characterized by bleeding due to the sloughing off of the uterine lining.

CHAPTER 16

Development

16.1 Embryonic Development

Gestation, the period of pregnancy, normally takes place over about nine months. Development before birth (prenatal development) begins with **fertilization**, the union of the sperm cell and female sex cell. Fertilization produces the **zygote**, or fertilized egg, in the oviduct. A series of events unfolds, producing the **embryo** (first two months) and **fetus** (last seven months).

The zygote begins to divide immediately to produce an early embryo by mitosis. The early stages of the embryo are: 2-cell, 4-cell, 8-cell, 16-cell, and 32-cell. This early division pattern is called **cleavage**, as the cell number increases without any increase in the cytoplasm. The 32-cell stage, for example, is the same size as the zygote.

Several days after fertilization, a mulberry-shaped mass, the **morula**, is formed in the oviduct. The morula develops into a **blastocyst**, a fluid-filled hollow ball of cells. This blastocyst will enter the uterus and implant in the endometrium at about 8 to 10 days after fertilization.

The early embryo changes from a hollow ball of cells through two processes: **morphogenesis** and **cell differentiation**. Morphogenesis is the movement of cells to establish a human outline. Cell differentiation means that cells specialize into different kinds. All cells descending from the zygote have a full complement of chromosomes and genes through mitosis. Depending on which genes are expressed in a group of cells, they specialize to become nerve cells, muscle cells, and so on.

Morphogenesis and cell differentiation establish three primary germ layers in the embryo by about two weeks after fertilization: the **ectoderm, mesoderm,** and **endoderm**. A continuation of these two processes in these germ layers form all future tissues and organs. Some examples are:

Ectoderm (outer layer) - Epidermis of skin, tooth enamel, lens and cornea of the eye, nervous system

Mesoderm (middle layer) - Dermis of skin, connective tissues, skeleton, skeletal muscles, circulatory system

Endoderm (inner layer) - Digestive tract and accessory organs, respiratory tract, kidney nephrons, bladder, several endocrine glands

Other significant events of embryonic development include:

Week 3 The embryo is surrounded by a membrane, the **amnion,** and amniotic fluid. The **placenta** starts to form.

Week 4 - The heart beats and is pumping blood. The limb buds form. The placenta is fully formed and working.

Week 6 - The limbs buds develop digits. A skeleton of cartilage forms.

Week 8 - All internal organs are produced. The embryo appears human-like.

Problem Solving Examples:

 What is meant by embryonic development? Describe the various stages of embryonic development.

A Embryonic development begins when an ovum is fertilized by a sperm and ends at parturition (birth). It is a process of change and growth that transforms a single-cell zygote into a multicellular organism.

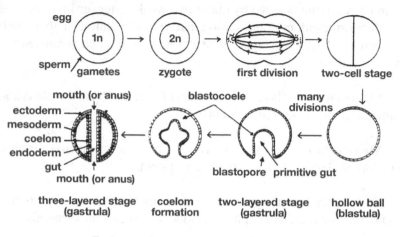

Early embryonic development in animals

The earliest stage of embryonic development is the one-celled, diploid zygote that results from the fertilization of an ovum by a sperm. Next is a period called cleavage, in which mitotic division of the zygote results in the formation of daughter cells called blastomeres. At each succeeding division, the blastomeres become smaller and smaller. When 16 or so blastomeres have formed, this solid ball of cells is called a morula. As the morula divides further, a fluid-filled cavity is formed in the center of the sphere, converting the morula into a hollow ball of cells called a blastula. The fluid-filled cavity is called the blastocoele. When cells of the blastula differentiate into two, and later three, embryonic germ layers, the blastula is called a gastrula. The gastrula period generally extends until the early forms of all major structures (e.g., the heart) are laid down. After this period, the developing organism is called a fetus. During the fetal period the various systems develop further. Though developmental changes in the fetal period are not as dramatic as those occurring during the earlier embryonic periods, they are extremely important.

Congenital defects may result from abnormal development during this period.

 Following fertilization, the zygote begins to cleave. Describe the processes the cells undergo through cleaving.

Cleavage cells are known as blastomeres. Blastomeres vary in size and content, principally by reason of differences in the amount, distribution, and other cytoplasmic inclusions they contain. The opposite side of the egg, an area where the nuclear material is located, is called the animal pole. In this case, the blastomeres nearer the animal pole tend to be smaller and are called micromeres. The cells near the vegetal pole, opposite the animal pole, are usually larger and are termed macromeres. As long as the entire egg divides into cells, the cleavage is said to be complete, or holoblastic. If the entire egg does not divide into cells, cleavage is incomplete and is confined to a small area that surrounds the animal pole. The rest of the egg remains uncleaved. Such incomplete cleavage is termed meroblastic.

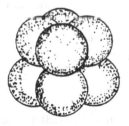 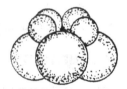

Radial and spiral cleavage patterns. Left: radial cleavage, charac-teristics of deuterostomes. The cells of the two layers are arranged directly above each other. Right: Spiral cleavage, characteristic of protosomes. The cells in the upper layer are located in the angles between the cells of the lower layer.

16.2 Fetal Development

Refinements of morphogenesis and differentiation produce the following results as the fetus develops.

Month 3 - The head is abnormally large when compared to the rest of the body. It is distinct with well-formed eyes and ears. The biological sex is identifiable by examining the external organs. Bone tissue gradually replaces the cartilage of the skeleton.

Month 4 - A bony skeleton is established. The skeletal muscles contract and produce body movements. The head is not as disproportionately large.

Month 5 - The internal organs continue to develop. The fetus may reach a weight of ¾ pound to 1 pound.

Month 6 - Fused eyelids begin to open. The fetus may reach a weight of 1.5 pounds.

Months 7 through 9 - There is a tremendous weight gain, with the fetus normally reaching 6 to 8 pounds by birth. The body length normally reaches 18 to 22 inches. The **fontanels**, soft membranous patches between the cranial plates, are distinct.

16.3 Parturition

Parturition is the process of birth. The fetus is expelled from the uterus and through the vagina by contractions of the myometrium.

Oxytocin, a hormone secreted from the posterior lobe of the pituitary gland, signals the uterus to develop the forceful contractions for birth. **Labor** begins when the uterus contracts approximately every 15 minutes. The length of each contraction during labor is over 30 seconds. The cervix dilates as the baby is born. The amnion may rupture, releasing the amniotic fluid through the vagina.

Shortly after the delivery of the baby, the placenta (afterbirth) passes through the vagina, pushed by uterine contractions.

Problem Solving Example:

Q What hormonal changes occur during the delivery of an infant (parturition)?

A Present theory holds that a shift in the balance of estrogen and progesterone is one important factor in parturition. Estrogen is known to stimulate contractions of the uterine muscles, and progesterone is known to inhibit muscular contraction. It is known that just before parturition, estrogen secretion by the placenta rises sharply, and this increase may play a role in the contraction of the uterus. It is therefore believed that, during pregnancy, progesterone suppresses contraction of the uterine muscles, but the rise of estrogen late in pregnancy overcomes the effects of the progesterone and initiates the contractions necessary for birth. Oxytocin, one of the hormones released from the posterior pituitary, is an extremely potent uterine muscle stimulant and is released as a result of stimulation of the hypothalamus by receptors in the cervix. Relaxin, a hormone secreted by the ovaries and placenta during pregnancy, is another hormone that may be important in parturition. Relaxin loosens the connections between the bones of the pelvis, thereby enlarging the birth canal to provide easier exit for the infant. Prostaglandins are fatty acid derivatives secreted by animal tissues. Prostaglandins stimulate the smooth muscle of many organs, including the smooth muscle of the wall of the uterus.

16.4 Postnatal Development

Development after birth, postnatal development, progresses over a series of stages: **infant**, **child**, **adolescent**, and **adult**.

Infant - For the first 24 months after birth, the infant develops many sensory and motor abilities. These abilities include focusing on objects as well as grasping and walking. Patterns of speech and language development unfold.

Child - Many emotional characteristics are established during this period. Physical growth is substantial. Refinements of mental capacities, such as reading, occur.

Adolescent - Beginning with the onset of puberty, this period begins with a substantial growth spurt. Behavioral changes occur as the individual begins to imitate adulthood. Many physiological changes occur with attainment of full adult stature, usually by the late teens.

Adult - Reached by about the age of 20, one's physical peak is usually attained in the early years of adulthood. Muscular strength and the ability to respond homeostatically, as examples, are optimal. The onset of aging is marked by a decrease in the number of functional cells in all organ systems. The rate of this decline, however, is extremely variable. Patterns of exercise and diet greatly influence the aging process.

Quiz: The Reproductive System and Development

1. During the human menstrual cycle, peak levels of estrogen and luteinizing hormone are associated with

    (A) the flow phase.

    (B) the early part of the follicular phase.

    (C) the latter part of the follicular phase.

    (D) the early part of the luteal phase.

    (E) the latter part of the luteal phase.

2. Luteinizing hormone (LH) and follicle stimulating hormone (FSH) are secreted by which gland?

    (A) Anterior pituitary

    (B) Posterior pituitary

    (C) Thyroid

    (D) Adrenal medulla

    (E) Adrenal cortex

3. Ovum and follicle development is stimulated by

    (A) increased FSH production.

    (B) low estrogen levels.

    (C) high estrogen levels.

    (D) high progesterone levels.

    (E) low progesterone levels.

4. During the proliferative phase of the female reproductive cycle, the pituitary increases secretion of

   (A) luteinizing hormone.

   (B) follicle stimulating hormone.

   (C) progesterone.

   (D) estrogen.

   (E) adrenocorticotropic hormone.

5. The stage during development in which there is a hollow ball of cells is called

   (A) blastulation.

   (B) morulation.

   (C) the isolecithal stage.

   (D) gastrulation.

   (E) ovulation.

6. The placenta originates from

   (A) embryonic cells.

   (B) maternal cells.

   (C) paternal cells.

   (D) Both (A) and (B).

   (E) Both (B) and (C).

7. The heart, bones, and blood develop primarily from the

   (A) endoderm.   (D) morula.

   (B) ectoderm.   (E) blastula.

   (C) mesoderm.

8. The period of gestation is divided into three trimesters. Which of the following events is correctly matched to its trimester of occurrence?

    (A) The third trimester is characterized by development and differentiation.

    (B) The greatest growth in size occurs in the first trimester.

    (C) The limb buds develop in the first trimester.

    (D) Kicking is felt by the mother in the first trimester.

    (E) Organ development begins in the second trimester.

9. What does NOT occur immediately after fertilization?

    (A) A sperm enters the outer membrane of the egg.

    (B) Cytoplasmic substances in the fertilized egg become rearranged.

    (C) The genetic material of the sperm and egg combine.

    (D) Cleavage occurs.

    (E) None of the above.

10. Gastrulation results in three primary tissue layers that give rise to all organs and tissues of the body. Which of the following statements is true?

    (A) Endoderm gives rise to muscle.

    (B) Epiderm gives rise to skin.

    (C) Mesoderm gives rise to bone.

    (D) Ectoderm gives rise to the gut lining.

    (E) Periderm gives rise to skin.

ANSWER KEY

1.	(C)	6.	(D)
2.	(A)	7.	(C)
3.	(A)	8.	(C)
4.	(B)	9.	(E)
5.	(A)	10.	(C)